Here's How to Treat Dementia

D1609454

WITHDRAWN

TOURO COLLEGE LIBRARY
Kings Hwy

Here's How Series

Thomas Murry, PhD
Series Editor

Here's How to Treat Childhood Apraxia of Speech by Margaret A. Fish

Here's How Children Learn Speech and Language: A Text on Different Learning Strategies by Margo Kinzer Courter

Here's How to Do Early Intervention for Speech and Language: Empowering Parents by Karyn Lewis Searcy

Here's How to Do Stuttering Therapy by Gary Rentschler

Here's How to Provide Intervention for Children with Autism Spectrum Disorder: A Balanced Approach by Catherine B. Zenko and Michelle Peters Hite

Here's How to Treat Dementia

Jennifer L. Loehr, MA, CCC-SLP
Megan L. Malone, MA, CCC-SLP

TOURO COLLEGE LIBRARY
Kings Hwy
WITHDRAWN

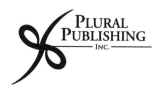

PLURAL
PUBLISHING
INC.

9194

KH

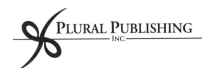

PLURAL PUBLISHING
INC.

5521 Ruffin Road
San Diego, CA 92123

e-mail: info@pluralpublishing.com
Website: http://www.pluralpublishing.com

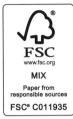

FSC
www.fsc.org
MIX
Paper from
responsible sources
FSC® C011935

Copyright © by Plural Publishing, Inc. 2014

Typeset in 11/15 Stone Informal by Flanagan's Publishing Services, Inc.
Printed in the United States of America by McNaughton & Gunn, Inc.

All rights, including that of translation, reserved. No part of this publication may be reproduced, stored in a retrieval system, or transmitted in any form or by any means, electronic, mechanical, recording, or otherwise, including photocopying, recording, taping, Web distribution, or information storage and retrieval systems without the prior written consent of the publisher.

For permission to use material from this text, contact us by
Telephone: (866) 758-7251
Fax: (888) 758-7255
e-mail: permissions@pluralpublishing.com

Every attempt has been made to contact the copyright holders for material originally printed in another source. If any have been inadvertently overlooked, the publishers will gladly make the necessary arrangements at the first opportunity.

Library of Congress Cataloging-in-Publication Data

Loehr, Jenny, author.
  Here's how to treat dementia / Jennifer L. Loehr, Megan L. Malone.
     p. ; cm. — (Here's how series)
  Includes bibliographical references and index.
  ISBN-13: 978-1-59756-448-9 (alk. paper)
  ISBN-10: 1-59756-448-6 (alk. paper)
  I. Malone, Megan L., author. II. Title. III. Series: Here's how series.
  [DNLM: 1. Dementia—rehabilitation. 2. Dementia—diagnosis. 3. Speech-Language Pathology—methods. WM 220]
  RC521
  616.8'3—dc23
                                                                        2013024779

10|3|19

Contents

Foreword

The "Here's How" series is a collection of texts that present a direct, "hands on" approach to understanding and treating a specific disorder. The series emanated out of an observation that speech-language pathologists who work in varied environments—hospitals, clinics, school systems, and private practices—attend workshops and clinical forums in large numbers at state and national meetings. Initially conceived as a series for beginning clinicians, we found that clinicians of all levels of training and experience were gravitating toward the "Here's How" series. In addition, teachers and students entering their initial off-campus placements were looking for materials that offered a "hands on" approach to various therapies. This series has covered topics including child language, autism, and fluency and literacy, just to name a few. This edition, *Here's How to Treat Dementia*, by Jennifer L. Loehr and Megan L. Malone, offers an in-depth approach to treating dementia.

The authors of *Here's How to Treat Dementia* are clinicians first and foremost with years of experience and success. The text includes the authors' well-documented and success-driven practices with the topics addressed. Clinicians will find practical information to raise their clinical practice to the next level and will enjoy sharing in the author's experiences, brought to life with case studies, case vignettes, and clinical tips.

Ms. Loehr and Ms. Malone address the importance of the types of memory that exist in dementia and how each of those memory systems diminishes in patients with dementia. They focus on the importance of initially treating the memory systems most resistant to decline then treating the systems that are necessary to daily function. The authors also emphasize the importance of treating aspects of non-declarative memory. Each chapter offers guidance as to how to achieve a network of memory functions that help patients with dementia retain related events and guide a patient through his or her day. The authors demonstrate how to improve the patient's awareness to the world around him/her and how to address specific needs of individuals based on the type of memory loss. While the clinician guides the treatment process and facilitates access to treatment, family members are encouraged to be involved in the treatment and support process. It is clear that Ms. Loehr and Ms. Malone have extensive experience with the treatment of dementia and, with this text, they share that experience with others. Clinicians and family members alike will each find the treatment guides valuable and easy to follow.

We hope you enjoy this and the other books in Plural Publishing's "Here's How" series.

Thomas Murry, PhD
Series Editor

Preface

This text is designed to serve as a sourcebook for speech-language pathologists (SLPs) and other rehabilitation professionals on how to effectively provide services to patients with dementia. It also is designed to help SLPs and other rehabilitation professionals work effectively with patients' families and caregivers. Both authors have worked with patients with dementia and their families and caregivers for a number of years, and it is our hope that this manual will provide easy-to-use and functional information to improve the therapy services and education to help these patients. Where possible, figures, example worksheets, and resource lists have been created to emphasize the main concepts of the text. These resources also may be found in the Appendix and may be reproduced for optimum functionality and use to improve the practice of all professionals working with not only patients with dementia but also their families, caregivers, and other care team members.

Part I of the book focuses on understanding dementia, from a basic understanding of how memory works to what causes dementia and understanding the current demographics of the disease, as well as common symptoms and physical considerations. The information provided in these chapters is not meant to be an exhaustive breakdown of dementia but instead was created to provide the treating professional with the most practical information on the disease in order to provide the best care for patients with dementia and to educate the patients' families and caregivers effectively on how dementia is defined and how it manifests itself in individuals diagnosed with it. Readers are encouraged to use this information as a springboard to complete further research on dementia in order to better understand it and treat it appropriately.

Part II of this text focuses on effective therapeutic interventions for dementia. Areas covered include dementia staging, evaluation tools and techniques, goal setting for patients with dementia, and current treatment trends. Because this book is a part of the "Here's How" series, this section of the book will likely be the most read and used in daily practice. The authors have focused heavily on providing the reader with the tools we have found the most useful in our own practices and have provided several examples of evaluation techniques, goal recommendations, and treatment techniques to help both new SLPs as well as more seasoned ones to work functionally and appropriately with patients with dementia. We hope that the examples provided will spark creativity in the reader to develop individualized goals and implement treatment that is tailored to each patient he/she serves.

Part III of the text examines additional considerations in treating individuals with dementia. This encompasses important areas such as patient and family education, documentation and reimbursement, dealing with behavioral issues, pharmacological intervention, treating the patient holistically, and special considerations for the home health SLP. Again, the authors have strived to include the most relevant and useful information on these topics as possible and encourage the reader to conduct his/her own individual research on these topics where applicable.

Final Notes from the Authors

This book was made possible through the efforts of many individuals. The work and research accomplished by the Myers Research Institute of Menorah Park Center for Senior Living in Beachwood, Ohio, inspired one of the authors, Megan Malone, to work in the field of dementia research and treatment. The mentorship and education provided by Dr. Cameron Camp, Dr. Rebecca Meehan, Dr. Marcia Neundorfer, and Dr. Jeanne Mattern has been instrumental in allowing this book to be produced. The dedicated staff of Myers Research, including Carole Kalman, Silvia Orsulic-Jeras, Gregg Gorzelle, Mike Skrajner, Vince Antenucci, Adena Joltin, and countless others also should be thanked for their numerous contributions to many of the ideas shared in this manual. The wonderful staff and residents of Menorah Park and Stone Gardens assisted living should be recognized for their participation in numerous research studies and projects throughout the years. The staff of HCR ManorCare, particularly Charles Batcher and Mary Casper, have been instrumental partners in participating in research studies and changing the face of dementia care on a national level. The staff of Gentiva Health Services in Akron, Ohio, also should be acknowledged for their dedication to serving older adults living with dementia in the home care environment and for allowing Ms. Malone to be an active team member in educating the staff in working effectively with persons with dementia and their families. Jenny Loehr was particularly inspired by the team of passionate professionals at Encompass Home Health. Bud Langham, PT. was inspirational in demonstrating that quality dementia programming isn't possible without the use of sound clinical judgment, evidenced based tools, and a desire to make a difference in the lives of those who suffer from dementia. The names of the talented co-workers and staff members, particularly SLPs, who we have worked with or who have taught us throughout the years are too many to count and too many to name here, but we thank you from the bottom of our hearts for your inspiration, support, and creativity.

To all readers of this text, welcome to this book! We thank you for allowing us to be a part of your practice and are hopeful that in some small part this text will help the millions of patients, families, and caregivers living with dementia to experience the best quality of care from caring and dedicated professionals, like you! Remember, "Persons with dementia live in the moment, so let's provide them with as many moments worth living as possible."

Acknowledgments

This work would not have been possible without the love and support of many individuals. Each author would like to separately acknowledge those whose unwavering support and inspiration have allowed this book to be created.

I would like to thank the following individuals whose love and support have not only made this book a reality but also my life a blessed, happy, and full one. You will never know how much you all mean to me! I love you and thank you all!

My parents, Charleen and Joseph Malone

My brothers, Brian and Craig

My sister-in-laws, Leann and Jessica

My nephews, Carter and Declan

My nieces, Alyssa and Nicole

My aunt and uncle, Susan and Bill Sparks

My cousins, Kelsey and Tim Sparks

My "sisters," Leah VanderKaay, Jill Sesplankis, Laura Kesterson, Susan Fraley, Shannon Constantine, and Sarah Russell

My inspirations, Estelle Campbell and Robertta Carothers

My co-author and partner-in-crime (and in fun!), Jenny Loehr

and

My patients, women and men, and their families who astound and inspire me daily to "keep up the good fight!"

—Megan L. Malone

There are many individuals whose influence and inspiration made it possible to put these words into print. Specifically, I would like to thank my father Jim, for always letting me know he believes in me, Linda for showing never-ending positive support, my husband Brian for loving me unconditionally, my son Jacob for always speaking out in my defense, and Josh for making me laugh every single day.

Thank you to the co-workers, family members, and caregivers who are "called" to do this work and who share the mission of dementia care. Special thanks to Megan who, through the years, has helped me see the work we do in a very positive, light-hearted way. I am so proud to work with you to spread the gospel of dementia care. This gig would have been a drag without you!

—Jenny L. Loehr

PART

I

Understanding Dementia

Part 1 of this book is divided into five chapters. Chapter 1 provides an overview for the speech-language pathologist (SLP) on how memory works in order to provide a greater understanding of how it is impacted when a person is diagnosed with dementia. Chapter 2 reviews the causes of dementia, including how dementia is diagnosed. Chapter 3 provides the demographics of dementia, including up-to-date statistics on this population and projections regarding care in the future. Chapter 4 focuses on the common symptoms of dementia and Chapter 5 discusses physical considerations, such as secondary diagnoses and comorbidities. These chapters serve to provide the SLP with a more in-depth understanding of dementia, which can serve as a foundation for developing treatment strategies and educating the families of these patients and the additional professionals caring for them.

1

How Memory Works

Memory is a complex system, made to be even more complex when we attempt to define and understand it. It is defined as "the mental faculty of retaining and recalling past experience based on the mental processes of learning, retention, recall, and recognition" (The American Heritage® Stedman's Medical Dictionary, 2007), but functionally our memory affects each and everything we do each and every day. This is why when it is damaged or affected by a disease, such as Alzheimer's, it can greatly impact how we live, what we do, and how we function. In order to better understand how speech-language pathologists (SLPs) can best treat persons living with dementia, it is important for us first to understand how memory works.

Memory Systems

In its simplest definition, memory is the running time line of what has happened in our lives. It stores the information of who we are and what we have done, along with the details of how to accomplish tasks, define and understand words, and function in the world. It was debated for some time if memory was in fact a singular system or if it actually is composed of a number of systems working together. Squire (2004) states that "memory is composed of multiple separate systems supported, for example, by the hippocampus and related structures, the amygdala, the neostriatum, and the cerebellum" and it is this idea that is the most widely accepted at this time (Eichenbaum & Cohen, 2001; Schacter, Wagner, & Buckner, 2000; Squire, Stark, & Clark, 2004). Squire (2004) discusses two main systems of memory: declarative memory and nondeclarative memory. These two systems make up what is known as long-term memory, which is where information is permanently stored (Mahendra & Apple, 2007). We focus our discussion on these two systems and their subsystems in order to glean a better understanding of how memory operates and is impacted by a diagnosis like dementia.

Declarative Memory

Declarative memory encompasses our everyday definition of memory. It refers to the capacity for conscious recollection about facts and events (Squire, 2004). Declarative memory, also known as explicit memory (daily learning of new information), can be divided into semantic memory (facts about the world) and episodic memory (the capacity to re-experience an event in the context in which it originally occurred) (Tulving, 1983). More specifically, "episodic memory refers to memory of events that a person has experienced in a specific place and at a particular time; whereas semantic memory refers to knowledge about the world that individuals share with other members of their culture, including the knowledge of a native language and facts learned in school" (Purves et al., 2008, p. 354). For example, recalling planting tulips in your garden last weekend would be an episodic memory, but knowing that tulips are perennial flowers would be categorized as a semantic memory. Often, episodic memories and semantic memories overlap to form what is known as autobiographical memory, which can be defined as memories of what occurs in our own lives (Purves et al., 2008). The hippocampus appears to be the structure at the center of processing new information that is encoded into memory, although lesions in other limbic areas also may result in problems with declarative memory (Goldman, 2000). Goldman (2000) also states that declarative memory incorporates other areas of memory including emotional memory, believed to be centered in the amygdala, which provides the emotional, more automatic feelings associated with a memory; working memory, the ability to hold new pieces of information in immediate memory, while manipulating other pieces of information, and lexical memory, which consists of specialized word knowledge, such as words as concepts and the phonemes making up these words (Mahendra & Apple, 2007; Schank, 1975). Figure 1–1 presents Squire's and Zola's (1996) taxonomy of long-term memory systems. See this figure to understand the neurological correlations of the subsystems of both declarative and nondeclarative memory.

When thinking of a person living with dementia, we often see information associated with declarative memory being more difficult to process and retrieve. Craik (2000) states that episodic memory is particularly vulnerable to the effects of aging and neurodegenerative disorders, like Alzheimer's disease (Craik, 2000). For example, we may see recent episodes in a person's life, such as what they ate for breakfast that morning, being very difficult to retrieve. General knowledge about the world and language also may be areas of difficulty over time. This is why we may see a person with dementia having trouble recalling certain facts, like a family member's name, or over time having increasing difficulty with expressing their wants and needs due to difficulty recalling the name of a certain object they want. These categories of information appear to be stored in areas supported by declarative memory and tend to be considered as areas of weakness or deficit in a person living with dementia. Sometimes, however, this information can be cued for retrieval by providing a semantic or phonemic cue to help "trigger the memory." For example, if a person is having difficulty recalling their daughter's name, we may try to "help" the person to the correct response by providing the first letter of the person's name (phonemic cue). ("Your daughter's name begins with the letter "M." Yes, her name is Mary.") An example of a semantic cue would be if a person was pointing at an apple

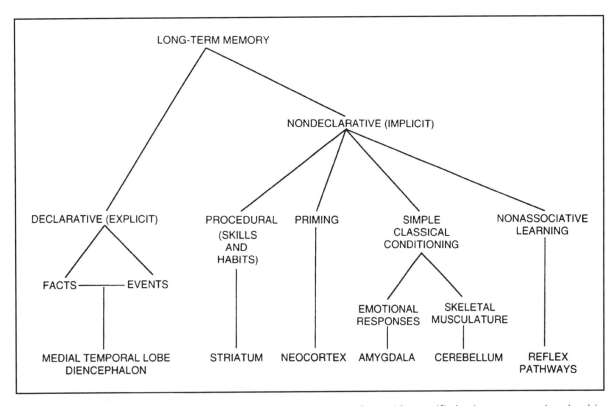

Figure 1–1. A taxonomy of long-term memory systems together with specific brain structures involved in each system. Adapted from "Structure and Function of Declarative and Nondeclarative Memory Systems," by L. R. Squire and S. M. Zola, November 26, 1996, *PNAS, 93*, 13515–13522. Copyright 1996 by the National Academy of Sciences, U.S.A.

but could not recall the word "apple" to indicate they wanted it. We may say, "It's red. It's a fruit. Your favorite pie is made of them. Yes, it's an apple." These types of cues often are used by SLPs to assist a person in recall of information, but these cues or the information associated with the cues often are not encoded into memory for later retrieval. This inability to learn and store information for later retrieval is a hallmark of the dementia diagnosis. Because dementia often is considered a progressive disorder when associated with diagnoses such as Alzheimer's, we may see persons who are in early stages of these disorders respond well to this type of cueing for retrieval of information, although the retrieval often is more effortful and over time will likely become more and more difficult for the person. We, as therapists, then must find ways to circumvent, or go around, these areas of weakness for our patients so that we can best support them through the stages of cognitive loss they likely are to experience. To best do this, we should focus our intervention efforts on the nondeclarative memory system.

Nondeclarative Memory

Nondeclarative memory, also known as implicit memory, has been found to be less impaired in persons with certain types of dementia (Brush & Camp, 1998). Mahendra and Apple (2007) state, "the specific neuropathology of Alzheimer's disease (AD) results in significant working and episodic memory impairments, but relatively spared nondeclarative memory." By definition, nondeclarative memory involves the ability to complete skills or habits without conscious recall of how to perform them. A distinction between declarative and nondeclarative memory is that declarative memory supports conscious recall of information, whereas nondeclarative memory does not afford awareness of any memory content (Squire & Zola, 1996). In other words, if declarative memory is considered to be the recall of "the what" (meaning, information), nondeclarative memory is considered to be the recall and performance of tasks or "the how." For example, a person who is able to recall the episode of playing the piano the previous day would be an example of a declarative memory skill ("the what"), whereas a person being able to sit down and actually play a song on the piano would be considered a nondeclarative memory task ("the how").

Nondeclarative memory includes:

- Memory for skills and habits: well-practiced, automatic routines, such as feeding yourself or getting dressed. These abilities may become more difficult for a person with dementia over time.

- Priming: increased sensitivity to stimuli after repeated exposures to that or related stimuli (Brush & Camp, 1998), similar to the idea of "practice makes perfect." The presence of priming in nondeclarative memory supports how a person can learn a new task and get better at completing it, the more they practice it. In a person with dementia, they may get increasingly better at locating their chair in the dining room of their assisted living facility by going there several times a day (priming), even though they have no conscious recollection of having gone there in the past (episodic memory).

- Procedural memory: supports learning of motor tasks and procedures (playing the piano, riding a bike) and development of cognitive skills (completing a puzzle) through repeated performance of the tasks. This includes recall of the ability to read printed material (Emery, 1999, 2003). If a person with dementia learned how to read during their lifetime and if the print is adjusted to meet the visual needs of the person, their ability to read and respond to the printed word can greatly help in compensating for their other memory deficits. This will be discussed further related to goals and treatment trends.

- Classical conditioning: "behaviors that are automatically produced in response to a particular set of stimuli" (Bayles & Tomoeda, 2007, p. 45). For example, learning that when you hear a fire alarm go off in a building, you should head to the nearest exit. In other words, a certain stimulus elicits a certain response. In a person with dementia, for example, the stimulus could be the therapist who works with them. If the person's therapy is going well and the patient is enjoying the experience, the patient could get up out of his seat and grab his walker upon seeing his therapist come down the hallway (stimulus = therapist; response = getting up to go to therapy), even if they have no conscious memory of who the therapist is or what they do in treatment. On the other hand, if the person is having a negative experience in therapy (not experiencing success, not learning or doing meaningful activities in treatment), the patient could instead pretend to fall asleep upon seeing the therapist come down the hallway or flat out refuse to go to treatment at all. Therefore, because this kind of learning and memory is possible in persons with dementia, it is very important for our therapy to be success oriented and meaningful to the patient.

- Non-associative learning: learning that there are not always significant associations between events. For example, if you move into a new home, the first few nights you may be awoken by the new sounds of the house and area around you. After a few nights, you learn that these sounds are insignificant and you are able to sleep through the night.

Please see Figure 1–1 for the visual representation of nondeclarative memory and its neurological correlations.

Applying Knowledge of the Memory Systems to Treatment

As stated earlier, it has been found that nondeclarative memory abilities are relatively spared in persons with dementia. This does not mean that there are not levels of impairment to these aspects of nondeclarative memory in a person over time. Table 1–1 outlines the impaired and spared aspects of memory through the progression of early-to-late stage Alzheimer's disease. Using this figure is helpful to the speech pathologist in the assessment of persons with dementia and in developing treatment plans for them. We discuss this further in later chapters, but a short overview now is helpful to our discussion of the memory systems.

Table 1–1 states that persons in the early stage of Alzheimer's are living with impairments in working and episodic memory but have relatively spared abilities in recognition

Table 1–1. Memory System Impairment in Stages of Alzheimer's Disease

	Early Stage AD	**Middle Stage AD**	**Late Stage AD**
Impaired systems	WM EM	WM EM SM (some impairment evident)	All of declarative memory
Relatively spared systems	Recognition memory SM NDM	Recognition memory SM (on recognition and cued recall tasks) NDM	Some aspects of NDM (habits, conditioned responses)

WM: Working Memory; *EM:* Episodic Memory; *SM:* Semantic Memory; *NDM:* Non-Declarative Memory.

Reprinted with permission from "Human Memory Systems: A Framework for Understanding Dementia," by N. Mahendra and A. Apple, November 27, 2007, *The ASHA Leader, 12*. Copyright 2007 by the American Speech-Language-Hearing Association. All rights reserved.

memory, semantic memory, and nondeclarative memory. This translates in treatment to *not* asking these persons questions related to facts and events ("What did you do today?" "What is your granddaughter's name?") because these questions attempt to tap into aspects of memory that are impaired in these individuals and can cause the person distress. Instead, it would be better to engage these individuals in tasks that allow for the use of their knowledge of procedures ("Would you help me fold the laundry?" "Please read the first sentence of the story aloud.") as these are considered to be abilities or strengths for them.

Table 1–1 also states that persons in the late stage of Alzheimer's disease have a great level of impairment in all aspects of declarative memory but still may exhibit aspects of nondeclarative memory, including habits and conditioned responses. This translates to treatment to the person possibly being unable to communicate verbally at all but still being able to perhaps shake someone's hand or respond to sensory stimuli, such as music or familiar scents.

As we continue our discussion of dementia through this manual, it is important for us to keep our focus on the many abilities and strengths of persons living with dementia. Much has been documented and discussed on the weaknesses and deficits of this population. We too cover these areas as part of further educating SLPs, but it is important to note, based on current research and the information shared here on impaired and relatively spared memory systems in dementia, that there indeed are many abilities that can be tapped into, even into the late stage of dementia. It is our job then as rehabilitation specialists to find those abilities and translate this research into functional activity, meaningful communication, and greater independence for our patients.

Please note: The intent of this chapter was to provide the rehabilitation clinician with a brief overview of memory and how it is impacted by the diagnosis of dementia. For more in-depth information on this topic, we suggest you further review the references listed at the end of the chapter.

Summary

- Memory is composed of a number of systems working together. These systems include both declarative and nondeclarative memory and their subsystems.

- Declarative memory, consisting of episodic, semantic, and lexical memory, has been found to experience greater impairment in persons with dementia. Therefore, the information stored in declarative memory tends to be harder to retrieve through the course of dementia.

- Nondeclarative memory, consisting of skills and habits, procedural memory, priming, classical conditioning, and non-associative learning, has been found to be relatively spared through the course of dementia. This is where our intervention and treatment efforts should be focused when working with this population.

- Although there are a number of weaknesses in the performance of cognitive and physical tasks as dementia progresses, there still are skills and abilities that remain that can help to guide treatment.

References

American Heritage® Stedman's Medical Dictionary The. (2007). Retrieved August 8, 2011, from DictionaryThe.com website at http://dictionary.reference.com/browse/memory

Bayles, K. A., & Tomoeda, C. K. (2007). *Cognitive–communication disorders of dementia.* San Diego, CA: Plural.

Brush, J., & Camp, C. (1998). *A therapy technique for improving memory: Spaced retrieval.* Beachwood, OH: Menorah Park Center for Senior Living.

Craik, F. I. M. (2000). Age-related changes in human memory. In D. C. Park & N. Schwarz (Eds.), *Cognitive aging: A primer* (pp. 75–92). Philadelphia, PA: Taylor and Francis.

Eichenbaum, H., & Cohen, N. J. (2001). *From conditioning to conscious recollection: Memory systems of the brain.* New York, NY: Oxford University Press.

Emery, V. O. B. (1999). On the relationship between memory and language in the dementia spectrum of depression, Alzheimer's syndrome, and normal aging. In H. Hamilton (Ed.), *Language and communication in old age: Multidisciplinary perspectives* (pp. 25–62). New York, NY: Garland.

Emery, V. O. B (2003). "Retrophylogenesis" of memory in dementia of the Alzheimer's type: A new evolutionary memory framework. In V. O. B. Emery & T. E. Oxman (Eds.), *Dementia: Presentations, differential diagnosis, and nosology* (pp. 177–238). Baltimore, MD: Johns Hopkins University Press.

Goldman, H. (2000). *Review of general psychiatry.* Columbus, OH: McGraw-Hill.

Mahendra, N., & Apple, A. (2007, November 27). Human memory systems: A framework for understanding dementia. *The ASHA Leader, 12.* Retrieved August 5, 2011, from http://www.asha.org/Publications/leader/2007/071127/f071127a/

Purves, D., Brannon, E., Cabeza, R., Huettel, S. A., LaBar, K., Platt, M. L., & Woldorff, M. (2008). *Principles of cognitive neuroscience.* Sunderdland, MA: Sinauer Associates.

Schacter, D. L., Wagner, A. D., & Buckner, R. L. (2000). Memory systems of 1999. In E. Tulving & F. I. M. Craik (Eds.), *Oxford handbook of memory* (pp. 627–643). New York, NY: Oxford University Press.

Schank, R. C. (1975). The structure of episodes in memory. In D. G. Bobrow and A. M. Collins (Eds.), *Representation and understanding: Studies in cognitive science.* New York, NY: Academic Press.

Squire, L. R. (2004). Memory systems of the brain: A brief history. *Neurobiology of Learning and Memory, 82,* 171–177.

Squire, L. R., & Zola, S. M. (1996, November 26). Structure and function of declarative and nondeclarative memory systems. *PNAS, 93,* 13515–13522.

Squire, L. R., Stark, C. E. L., & Clark, R. E. (2004). The medial temporal lobe. *Annual Review of Neuroscience, 27,* 279–306.

Tulving, E. (1983). *Elements of episodic memory.* Cambridge, MA: Oxford University Press.

CHAPTER

2

What Causes Dementia?

The answer to the question, "What causes dementia?" is unanswerable. There are multiple types of dementia and multiple genetic and environmental factors that may cause dementia. In order to understand the causes of dementia, it is important to understand the true definition of dementia. The medical community has misused the word or term "dementia" for decades. Physicians have been known to use this diagnosis randomly as a patient demonstrates symptoms of forgetfulness or general cognitive loss. Unfortunately, the error in labeling patients with dementia without proper evaluation can curtail necessary and appropriate pharmacological and therapeutic intervention. It is important to understand that dementia is not a diagnosis in of itself. This chapter explores more about what dementia really is. The expectation is not that you will have all of the answers, however, the expectation is that you will feel a little more empowered by having the facts.

Dementia refers to a group of symptoms caused by changes in the brain. These changes are a result of nerve cell damage affecting the transmission of nerve impulses or the communication pathways of the brain. The hallmark symptom of dementia is memory loss, but other cognitive, behavioral, and personality changes can occur as well. It also is important to know that just because someone suffers from memory loss does not mean there is dementia. Illness, injury, dehydration, and depression are only a few reasons that cause changes in the brain. With proper diagnosis and treatment, some of the causes are reversible.

The two key principles that underlie the concept of dementia are: (1) the affected person has experienced a decline from some previously higher level of functioning, and (2) the dementia "significantly" interferes with work or usual social activities (Knopman, Bradley, & Peterson, 2003). So, a patient who suffers a change in condition, a decline in thinking or memory during a period of time fits into this dementia category. This change in thinking can include the ability to follow and understand directions, remembering names or appointments, language deficits, or the ability to make good decisions. In addition, the patient whose cognitive deficits interfere with the execution of activities of daily living. Further explanation is provided in the following chapters.

How Is Dementia Diagnosed?

It takes more than only a quick checkup at the general physician's office to get an official diagnosis of dementia. We frequently see patients given a dementia diagnosis from their doctor because they have been a little forgetful or have an unexplained decline in mental status. This method of diagnosis is not complete and is a disservice to the patient.

To properly diagnose the etiology causing these symptoms, a physician must obtain a thorough patient history, assess function of daily activities, and administer and interpret the appropriate neurological and mental status evaluations. Physicians commonly refer to the criteria given in the *Diagnostic and Statistical Manual of Mental Disorders,* Fourth Edition (DSM-IV, 1994). This manual is used to help medical professionals make diagnosis by matching the symptoms listed for each diagnosis. To meet DSM-IV criteria of dementia, the following are required:

1. Symptoms must include decline in memory and in at least one of the following cognitive abilities: (a) Ability to generate coherent speech or understand written language; (b) Ability to recognize or identify objects, assuming intact sensory function; (c) Ability to execute motor activities, assuming intact motor abilities, sensory function, and comprehension of the required task; and (d) Ability to think abstractly, make sound judgments, and carry out complex tasks.

2. The decline in cognitive abilities must be severe enough to interfere with daily life. (DSM-IV, 1994)

Taking this information from the DSM-IV, the criteria can be broken down into four areas of cognition and/or language called domain criteria:

1. Recent memory: The ability to learn, retain, and retrieve newly acquired information (i.e., ability to remember what one had for a previous meal or recalling going to a movie the evening before last).

2. Language: The ability to comprehend and express verbal information (i.e., increased word finding problems).

3. Visuospatial function: The ability to manipulate and synthesize nonverbal, geographic, or graphic information (i.e., demonstrating increased falls due to poor depth perception).

4. Executive function: The ability to perform abstract reasoning, solve problems, plan for future events, mentally manipulate more than one idea at a time, maintain mental focus in the face of distraction, or shift mental effort easily (Knopman et al., 2003) (i.e., this may affect many activities of daily living including cooking, driving, paying bills, etc.).

As soon as the physician suspects a decline in cognition and matching criteria in the DSM-IV, further physical evaluation of the patient is conducted such as blood and urine sampling to detect common medical problems found in elderly individuals including but not limited to metabolic disorders, vitamin deficiencies, or infections. Unfortunately, these issues are very common in the elderly and also can cause altered mental status that mirrors dementia. Misdiagnosis can lead to serious illness and possibly death. In some instances, further investigation through brain imaging such as MRI may provide a fuller view of the brain, helping the physician in identifying pathology such as tumors, lesions, or vascular impairment.

By determining the probable cause, reversible dementia often can be identified and treated. However, most types of dementia are nonreversible (degenerative). Nonreversible means the changes in the brain that are causing the dementia cannot be stopped or turned back. It is important to get the earliest and most accurate diagnosis in order to allow patients and caregivers time to adjust, prepare, and adapt a lifestyle that will ensure optimal safety and well-being.

Classifications

Dementia disorders can be classified many different ways. Disorders can be classified into different groups that share common features and parts of the brain that are affected. Some types of dementia fit into more than one of these classifications. According to the National Institute of Neurological Disorders and Stroke and the National Institute of Health, the following are common classifications:

Cortical dementia: Dementia where the brain damage affects the brain's cortex, or outer layer. Cortical dementias tend to cause problems with memory, language, thinking, and social behavior.

Subcortical dementia: Dementia that affects parts of the brain below the cortex. Subcortical dementia tends to cause changes in emotions and movement, in addition to problems with memory.

Progressive dementia: Dementia that gets worse over time, gradually interfering with more and more cognitive abilities.

Primary dementia: Dementia such as Alzheimer's dementia that does not result from any other disease.

Secondary dementia: Dementia that occurs as a result of a physical disease or injury. Examples include Parkinson's disease, Multiple Sclerosis, and normal pressure hydrocephalus (NPH) (National Institute of Neurological Disorders and Stroke (NINDS), 2011).

Common Diagnoses

Alzheimer's Disease

Alzheimer's disease (AD) is the most common cause of dementia in people aged 65 and older. Recent statistics published by the National Alzheimer's Association indicate that four million people in the United States currently are living with the disease; one in ten people are over the age of 65, and nearly half of those over 85 have AD (Alzheimer's Association, 2011).

There are volumes of journals and text books written about Alzheimer's dementia. It is Alzheimer's disease so we are going to keep it as simple as possible so that you can impart this information to your patients and family members. AD is characterized by two abnormalities in the brain. Amyloid plaques and neurofibrillary tangles. The development of these plaques and tangles interrupt the neuronal transport system in the brain, impairing communication between nerve cells, causing the brain to atrophy or die. Patients in early stages of AD may experience memory impairment, lapses of judgment, and subtle changes in personality. As the disease progresses, memory and language problems worsen, affecting the functioning of activities of daily living such as managing finances and medication management. These patients may easily become disoriented and confused in new or unfamiliar surroundings. During the later stages of the disease, patients may suffer worsening motor control functions including bowel/bladder control and swallowing that most often leads to aspiration pneumonia. It is common for patients to lose the ability to verbally communicate or identify and recognize family members. On average, patients with AD live for eight to ten years after diagnosis (Alzheimer's Association, 2011).

Vascular Dementia

This is the second most common cause of dementia. It accounts for up to 20 percent of all dementias and is caused by brain damage from cardiovascular problems—usually strokes. It also may coexist with AD. The incidence of vascular dementia increases with advancing age and is similar in men and women.

Symptoms of vascular dementia often begin suddenly. Patients may have a history of high blood pressure, vascular disease, heart attacks, or strokes. This disease may or may not get worse with time depending on whether or not the patient suffers additional strokes. This type of dementia mirrors that of AD except that patients with vascular dementia do not suffer personality changes and maintain normal levels of emotional responsiveness until later stages of the disease. People with vascular dementia often wander at night and often have other problems commonly found in people who have had stroke, including depression and incontinence.

There are several types of vascular dementia. The most common is called multi-infarct dementia (MID). This is caused by numerous small strokes in the brain. The symptoms of MID often are limited to one side of the body or may affect only one or a few specific functions such as language. These are called "local" or "focal" symptoms as opposed to "global" symptoms seen in AD (NINDS, 2011).

Lewy Body Dementia

Lewy body dementia (LBD) is the most common of the progressive types of dementia. In LBD, cells die in the brain's cortex, or outer layer, and in a part of the mid-brain. Many of the remaining nerve cells contain abnormal structures called Lewy bodies that are the hallmark of the disease. These Lewy bodies contain a protein that is similar to that found in patients who suffer from Parkinson's disease. The cognitive symptoms of LBD mirror AD and may include memory impairment, poor judgment, and confusion. Typically, patients with LBD also suffer from visual hallucinations, Parkinsonian symptoms such as shuffling gait and flexed posture, and a day-to-day fluctuation in the severity of symptoms. Patients with LBD live on average seven years after symptoms begin (Lewy Body Dementia Association, 2011).

Frontal Temporal Dementia

Frontal temporal dementia (FTD) sometimes is referred to as frontal lobe dementia because it describes atrophying of the nerve cells found in the frontal or temporal lobes of the brain. Experts believe FTD accounts for 2 to 10% of all cases of dementia. Symptoms of FTD appear between the ages of 40 and 65 with most patients having a family history of dementia suggesting a genetic factor in the disease. Patients with FTD live on average, from five to ten years after diagnosis.

Due to the structures found in the frontal and temporal lobes of the brain that control judgment and social behavior, people with FTD often have problems socially interacting with other people. They may exhibit impolite or socially inappropriate behaviors. They may have impulsive, compulsive, or repetitive behaviors such as stealing or overeating. Other common symptoms include speech and language deficits and motor problems affecting balance. Memory loss can occur but typically will present late in the progression of the disease.

The most common types of FTD are Pick's disease and primary progressive aphasia (PPA). Pick's disease generally runs in families and is likely due to faulty genes. This disease usually begins after age 50 and causes changes in personality and behavior that gradually worsens over time. PPA can occur in people early in their forties. Receptive and/ or expressive aphasia is the hallmark of this disease with a gradual progression over time. As the disease progresses, memory and attention also may be impaired and patients may show personality and behavioral changes. Many but not all people with PPA develop symptoms of dementia (NINDS, 2011).

Korsakoff's Syndrome

This brain disorder usually is associated with heavy alcohol consumption during a long period of time. This syndrome is caused by lack of thiamine (vitamin B1), which affects the brain and nervous system. Thiamine deficiency often is seen in people who consume excessive amounts of alcohol. Those affected tend to be men between the ages of 45 and 65 with a long history of alcohol misuse, though it is possible to have Korsakoff's syndrome at an older or younger age. The main symptom is memory loss, particularly of events arising after the onset of the condition. Other symptoms may include difficulty in acquiring new information or learning new skills, change in personality, lack of insight into the condition, and confabulation (Alzheimer's Association, 2011).

HIV-Associated Dementia

HIV-associated dementia (HAD) results from infection with the human immunodeficiency virus (HIV) that causes AIDS. HAD can cause widespread destruction of the brain's white matter. This leads to a type of dementia that generally includes impaired memory, apathy, social withdrawal, and difficulty concentrating. People with HAD often develop movement problems as well. There is no specific treatment for HAD, but AIDS drugs can delay onset of the disease and may help to reduce symptoms (NINDS, 2011).

Huntington's Disease

Huntington's disease (HD) is a hereditary disorder caused by a faulty gene. The children of people with the disorder have a 50% chance of inheriting the gene, and everyone who inherits it will eventually develop the disorder. The onset of symptoms varies with this disease. Symptoms of HD include involuntary movements such as twitches and muscle spasms, problems with balance and coordination, personality changes such as irritability, depression and mood swings, and trouble with memory, concentration, or making decisions. There currently is no cure for HD, but research on potential treatments is accelerating since scientists identified the gene involved (NINDS, 2011).

Normal Pressure Hydrocephalus

Normal pressure hydrocephalus (NPH) is an abnormal increase of cerebrospinal fluid (CSF) in the brain's ventricles or cavities. Although it is not one of the more common diagnoses, it is good to know about this disorder because early detection can result in nearly full reversal of cognitive deficits. NPH occurs if the normal flow of CSF throughout the brain and spinal cord is blocked in some way. This causes the ventricles to enlarge, putting pressure on the brain. NPH can occur in people of any age but is most common in the elderly population. It may result from a subarachnoid hemorrhage, head trauma, infection, tumor, or complications of surgery. Symptoms of NPH include progressive mental impairment and dementia, problems with walking, and impaired bladder control, leading to urinary frequency and/or incontinence. Treatment for NPH involves surgical placement of a shunt in the brain to drain excess CSF into the abdomen where it can be absorbed. This allows the brain ventricles to return to their normal size. As stated previously, early diagnosis and treatment is important and improves the chance of a good recovery (NINDS, 2011).

Dementia Pugilistica

Dementia pugilistica, also called chronic traumatic encephalopathy or "Punch Drunk Syndrome," is caused by head trauma, such as that experienced by people who have been punched many times in the head during boxing, playing football, or ice hockey. The most common symptoms of the condition are dementia and parkinsonism, which can appear many years after the trauma occurs. Affected individuals also may develop poor coordination, gait ataxia, impaired hearing, tremors, and slurred speech (Pineda & Gould, 2010).

Corticobasal Degeneration

Corticobasal degeneration (CBD) is a progressive disorder characterized by nerve cell loss and atrophy of multiple areas of the brain. Initial symptoms, which begin at or around age 60, may first appear on one side of the body but eventually will affect both sides. Some of the symptoms such as poor coordination and rigidity are similar to those found in Parkinson's disease. Other symptoms may include memory loss, visual-spatial problems, apraxia, and dysphagia. Death often is caused by pneumonia or other secondary problems such as sepsis or pulmonary embolism (NINDS, 2011).

Other Conditions Causing Dementia

There are a multitude of other conditions that can cause dementia or dementia-like symptoms. It is good for the SLP to be aware of these conditions as you may be able to assist in detection and reversal of the dementia symptoms. It is important to clarify that your job as the SLP in NOT to make a diagnosis. If you suspect any of the following conditions, it is very appropriate to alert the patient and/or family member and suggest they see their physician:

Nutritional deficiencies

Infections

Subdural hematomas

Poisoning

Anoxia

Brain Tumors

Metabolic changes

Vitamin B12 deficiency

Chronic alcohol abuse

Depression

Medication-induced dementia (NINDS, 2011).

What Is Not Dementia?

There are a few conditions that cause symptoms similar to that of dementia but are not considered to be dementia. We thought it would be good to add this section as it is good information to share with the lay community and dispel many of the dementia-related myths that are common today:

Age-related cognitive decline is not dementia. As people age, they may experience slow processing and mild memory impairment. These occurrences are normal and not considered to be dementia. It is good to spread this positive message. People should not expect to get dementia just because they live to be old.

Mild cognitive impairment is not dementia. It is similar to that of age-related cognitive decline as it presents as memory impairment and processing issues that are not severe enough to be classified as dementia. The folks who suffer from mild cognitive impairment are the people you sit next to in church who tell you the same story each week, who occasionally forget where they parked the car at the grocery store, or who mix up the names of their children and grandchildren. They still are functioning fairly normally, having developed coping strategies and compensatory measures, and their mental status remains stable.

Depression is not dementia. Depression is an illness that causes a patient to appear unresponsive, passive, slow, confused, and forgetful. This condition is the most misdiagnosed illness in the elderly as the symptoms easily mimic that of dementia and deserves some extra focus in this chapter. Depressive disorder is not a normal part of aging. Emotional experiences of sadness, grief, response to loss, and temporary "blue" moods are normal. Persistent depression that interferes significantly with ability to function is not. Health professionals mistakenly may think that persistent depression is an acceptable response to other serious illnesses and the social and financial hardships that often accompany aging—an attitude often shared by older people themselves. This contributes to low rates of detection, diagnosis, and treatment in older adults. If you suspect your patient is suffering from depression (remember you are not the one diagnosing!), it would be helpful to encourage and be a part of your patient pursuing treatment. It even may be beneficial to do a little background detective work and look into how long the depressive symptoms have been present. You may find in your investigation that the symptoms coincided with a life-altering event (i.e., death of a spouse, transition from home to a facility, etc.) and that similarly, the depressive symptoms also coincided with the onset of symptoms of dementia. This information would be very helpful if provided to the medical professional who would be diagnosing and treating the depression.

Conclusion

As the population ages, it is important to dispel the myth that cognitive decline is a normal occurrence. As illustrated above, there are a multitude of common diseases and illnesses that can lead to symptoms of dementia. The rapid population growth and the advent of baby boomers reaching the age of 65 during this decade will no doubt reveal an increase in patients that will need appropriate diagnoses and treatment. With adequate diagnosis, the clinician will be able to build and facilitate the appropriate treatment plan necessary to help these patients reach and maintain a level of functioning and overall health and well-being for many years into their diagnosis.

References

Alzheimer's Association. (2011). Alzheimer's disease facts and figures. *Alzheimer's & Dementia: The Journal of the Alzheimer's Association, 7*(2).

American Psychiatric Association. (1994). *Diagnostic and statistical manual of mental disorders (DSM-IV)* (4th ed.). Washington, DC: Author.

Knopman, D. S., Bradley, B. F., & Peterson, R. C. (2003). Essentials of the proper diagnoses of mild cognitive impairment, dementia, and major subtypes of dementia. *Mayo Clinic Proceedings, 10*(78), 1290–1308. Retrieved February 15, 2013, from http://www.mayoclinic proceedings.com

Lewy Body Dementia Association. (2011). *Understanding Lewy body dementia.* Retrieved February 10, 2013, from http://www.lbda. org/node/199#Understanding_LBD

National Institute of Neurological Disorders and Stroke (NINDS). (2011). *The dementias: Hope through research.* Retrieved February 10, 2013, from http://www.ninds.nih.gov/de mentias/detail_dementia.htm

Pineda, P., & Gould, D. (2010). The neuroanatomical relationship of dementia pugilistica and Alzheimer's disease. *Neuroanatomy, 9,* 5–7. Retrieved February 10, 2013, from http:// www.neuroanatomy.org/2010/005_007.pdf

3

Demographics of Dementia

Why Do We Need to Understand the Demographics of Dementia?

As speech-language pathologists (SLPs), it is important not only to understand the disease processes we treat but also to understand how these diseases are broken down in the population and what is projected for care and treatment of them in the future. This not only allows us to be more well-informed clinicians but also allows us to better educate the patients, families, and caregivers we work with on a daily basis. This chapter will focus on the current statistics of dementia . . . who is affected and what are the projected treatment trends, along with providing the SLP with an understanding of how to interpret and use the data reported by agencies, such as the Centers for Disease Control and the National Alzheimer's Association, in order to maximize our understanding of dementia and our ability to educate others (our patients, their caregivers, and other professionals) in what presently is happening with understanding the disease and what the future may hold for it.

What Does the Face of Dementia Look Like?

Age

To put it simply, we are living longer. Advances in health care, a focus on improved quality of life, and overall healthier lifestyles are shifting the lifespan to ages older than ever seen before. The Centers for Disease Control (CDC) reports that the number of people aged 65 years and older is expected to increase from 35 million in 2000 to 71 million in 2030. The number of people aged 80 years and older also is expected to double, from 9.3 million in 2000 to 19.5 million in 2030 (Chapman, Williams, Strine, Anda, & Moore, 2006). Chapman and the Centers for Disease Control also report the findings of Hendrie (1998) and Ebly (1994) that the prevalence of dementia has been estimated to be approximately 6% to 10% of individuals aged 65 years or older; prevalence increases with age, rising from 1% to 2% among those aged 65 to 74 to 30% or more of those aged 85 or older (Hendrie, 1998). Forty percent of those ages 90 to 94 were reported to suffer from dementia, with the prevalence of dementia peaking at 58% among individuals older than 94 years (Ebly, Parhad, Hogan, & Fung, 1994). It is important to note that currently a majority of older adults do not exhibit dementia and that these statistics do not include the adults who are under 65 years of age living with early onset dementia. The Alzheimer's Association reports that approximately 4% of the 5.4 million Americans with Alzheimer's have early onset and that these people typically are in their 40s and 50s (Alzheimer's Association, 2012b). Overall, however, the face of dementia tends to be one of a person over 65 years of age, and that because our population is living longer, dementia will continue to be a growing public health concern.

Race and Gender

It is estimated that more women than men are living with Alzheimer's or other dementias. The Alzheimer's Association (2012) reports that two-thirds of Americans living with Alzheimer's disease (AD) are women. Of the 5.2 million people aged older than 65 years with AD in the United States, 3.4 million are women, and 1.8 million are men. This primarily is explained by the fact that women tend to live longer than men.

Years of education also appears to be a factor in the risk for developing Alzheimer's or other dementias. Those who are considered to have fewer years of education have been found to be at a higher risk for developing dementia. Researchers believe that those with higher levels of education may be able to compensate better for cognitive changes in the brain related to dementia and also have better access to health care, resulting in better overall health in general than those people with less education and in lower socio-economic groups (Alzheimer's Association, 2012a).

It is reported that most people living with Alzheimer's in the United States primarily are white and non-Hispanic. However, it has been found that older African Americans and Hispanics are much more likely to develop Alzheimer's and other dementias. Older African Americans are twice as likely as older white persons to have AD and other dementias, while Hispanics are 1.5 times more likely than their white counterparts (Alzheimer's Association, 2012a). There are many possible reasons for these differences in prevalence, including genetic factors specific to race (African American and Hispanic populations tend to have an increased prevalence of both high blood pressure and diabetes) and lower levels of education. It also is reported that missed diagnosis of dementia is more common among non-white populations, which is a growing concern as these populations are estimated to increase in the future, resulting in more people living with the symptoms of AD and dementia and not receiving proper treatment due to non-diagnosis.

Does Where You Live Matter?

Researchers have analyzed regions of the United States and have projected the number of persons living with Alzheimer's disease living in these areas by the year 2025. Data from Hebert (2004) compiled by the Alzheimer's Association shows that by 2025, states in the South and West will likely experience a doubling or greater of persons with Alzheimer's disease, while states such as Alaska and Colorado will experience increases of at least 50%. This is explained by the growing number of persons aged 65 and over living in these areas (Herbert, et. al, 2004). It is important to note that this information does not mean that because you live in these states, you have a greater risk of developing dementia. However, it does have a large impact on the health care and management of the disease in these areas and an increased need for caregiver education in these areas in the future to help care for these individuals.

What About the Caregivers?

It is estimated that nearly 15 million Americans provide unpaid caregiving services to people living with dementia (Alzheimer's Association, 2012a). These caregivers typically are family members but also can be friends and other relatives. The stress and burden of providing care to persons living at home with dementia has been well documented. The physical and emotional demands are often taxing, and financial strain also can be experienced in the ongoing care of these individuals. It is becoming increasingly important for the care of the caregiver to be a priority to healthcare providers not only to assist in the care and advocacy of the person with dementia but also to maintain overall health and well-being of those who care for them.

Paid caregivers, such as home health aides, nursing assistants, and professional caregivers, also comprise a large number of persons caring for persons with dementia in their homes or in facility settings. These caregivers provide similar assistance to unpaid caregivers, such as assistance with activities of daily living (bathing, dressing, eating/meal preparation) and household chores/tasks. Many of these professionals receive training in how to effectively work with the dementia population, but this education typically is limited and often is learned "on the job" with the patients they assist. The need for continued education and support of all caregivers, both paid and unpaid, is paramount to the quality of care individuals with dementia receive. It is important, then, for professionals with a skilled knowledge of dementia and how to work with individuals with the diagnosis, like SLPs, to provide ongoing education to the caregiver. We will look at caregiver education more in depth in Chapter 10 of this manual.

What Do the Stats Say About the Future?

Looking into the crystal ball and trying to predict the future for those living with dementia, those caring for these individuals, and all of us who are aging may look somewhat bleak by simply looking at the statistics. However, there are advances in understanding this disease and how to treat it occurring on a daily basis. The important thing to remember is that even though the data points to the prevalence of this disease and the cost of managing it is only going to increase in the future, our current understanding of its onset and prevention of dementia is improving.

As professionals working with this population, it is of the upmost importance that we continue to educate ourselves on the prevention, diagnosis, and treatment trends being researched and reported by credible researchers, associations, and government agencies. It is part of our scope of practice to provide resources to our patients and their caregivers to build their understanding of dementia and how best to deal with it in their daily lives. The statistics reported in this manual and in other sources are important but do not provide enough to help the individuals we serve in understanding what is happening to them or their loved ones. Therefore, it should be cautioned that while sharing statistics like the ones mentioned in this chapter can paint a picture of how the disease projects itself on our population and how it will affect us all in the future, it is by no means enough when it comes to educating and comforting the people we serve. This information can be scary when presented without explanation. Many of our patients or caregivers will do their own research on dementia, typically on the internet, where the information can be inaccurate, incomplete, or without supporting evidence. Again, it is up to us and other professionals working with persons with dementia and their families to provide accurate, complete, and validated information to help build understanding, acceptance, and the ability for all of us to best care for this population. A list of resources/agencies is provided at the end of this manual for you to use in your ongoing education about dementia and other aging-related issues ("Dementia Resource List"). This list can be copied and reproduced to provide to families and other professionals during in-service or marketing presentations. Along with this list is a "Dementia Fact Sheet" summarizing the statistics outlined in this chapter. Again, these data are not presented to scare people but to provide a better understanding of how dementia currently is affecting our population. They should not only be shared but also explained in order to reduce the already present fear and anxiety associated with a dementia diagnosis.

This information also can be helpful to the SLP working in any setting with older adults to promote a need for skilled services from a speech therapist. It can be presented to physicians, rehabilitation managers, and other healthcare professionals to show the need for patients and caregivers to receive speech therapy services to increase ability, safety, quality of life, and assist in the reduction of caregiver burden.

Summary

- Dementia typically affects adults aged 65 and older. The prevalence of dementia is projected to increase in the future due to the increasing lifespan of the population.
- Dementia is more prevalent in women than in men, primarily due to the fact that women live longer.

- Years of education appears to impact a person's risk for developing Alzheimer's disease and related dementias. Typically, persons with more years of education are better able to compensate for cognitive changes and have better access to health care.

- A majority of the persons living with Alzheimer's disease in the United States are white and non-Hispanic. However, older adults who are African American or Hispanic have a higher risk of developing dementia due to genetic and health factors, such as increased risk of high blood pressure and diabetes, reduced levels of education, and sometimes limited access to health care.

- It is estimated that the prevalence of Alzheimer's disease will increase in the coming years. By 2025 in the United States, states in the South and West are likely to see the largest increases in persons with dementia due to the amount of older adults projected to be living in those areas at that time.

- Nearly 15 million people in the United States are acting as nonpaid caregivers to persons with dementia. Caregiver stress and burden is an ongoing concern and area of focus for professionals working with the dementia population. Paid caregivers also provide many services to persons with dementia, both in homes and facility settings. Ongoing education for both paid and unpaid caregivers on understanding dementia and managing it effectively should be an area of focus for healthcare professionals.

- The future for dementia may look grim according to the statistics, but new advances and research are ongoing. Speech therapists and other professionals working with this population and their families have a responsibility to remain updated on the latest findings and treatments, interpret the results and findings accurately, and provide resources to allow for the best quality of care for these patients.

References

Alzheimer's Association. (2012a). Alzheimer's disease facts and figures. *Alzheimer's & Dementia: The Journal of the Alzheimer's Association, 8*, 131–168.

Alzheimer's Association. (2012b). Younger/early onset Alzheimer's and dementia. Retrieved from http://www.alz.org/alzheimers_disease_early_onset.asp

Chapman, D. P., Williams, S. M., Strine, T. W., Anda, R. F., & Moore, M. J. (2006). Dementia and its implications for public health. *Prev Chronic Dis [serial online]*. Retrieved June 30, 2013, from http://www.cdc.gov/pcd/issues/2006/apr/pdf/05_0167.pdf

Ebly, E. M., Parhad, I. M., Hogan, D. B., & Fung, T. S. (1994). Prevalence and types of dementia in the very old: Results from the Canadian Study of Health and Aging. *Neurology, 44*, 1593–1600.

Hebert, L. E., Scherr, P. A., Bienias, J. L., Bennett, D. A., & Evans, D. A. (2004). State-specific projections through 2025 of Alzheimer's disease prevalence. *Neurology, 62*(9), 1645.

Hendrie, H. C. (1998). Epidemiology of dementia and Alzheimer's disease. *American Journal of Geriatric Psychiatry, 6*, S3–S18.

CHAPTER

4

Common Symptoms of Dementia

Introduction

In looking at symptoms of dementia, it is important to keep the definition of dementia in the back of your mind. You will recall that the definition of dementia is a set of symptoms caused by an illness or disease process affecting the brain. The symptoms and their severity will vary depending on the cause of the dementia and how far the disease has progressed. Of course, it is important to note that no two demented patients are alike and there are many other factors such as the environment, age, medical complications, and comorbidities that will affect the severity of the symptoms. In most cases, the symptom characteristics and their severity follow a similar pattern among dementia diagnoses.

In this chapter, we discuss some of the most common characteristics that are manifestations of dementia. We also will look into some of the more common disease processes that cause dementia and point out some of the hallmark symptom characteristics that help us differentiate between the different diseases.

Most Common Symptoms

The essential feature of dementia is the development of cognitive deficits that affect normal daily functioning and socialization. The *Diagnostic and Statistical Manual of Mental Disorders,* Fourth Edition (DSM-IV-TR) reveals that in order to have a true diagnosis of dementia, there will be multiple cognitive deficits that include memory impairment and at least one other cognitive component (American Psychiatric Association, 2000). A diagnosis of dementia cannot be made if only one cognitive deficit presents itself independently of any other cognitive deficits. Furthermore, these deficits must show a progression from a previously higher level of functioning (American Psychiatric Association, 2000). To begin, we will look at the most prominent areas of cognitive functioning.

Memory Impairment

Memory loss appears to be the hallmark of most of the common dementias. The Alzheimer's Association lists memory impairment as the first 'warning sign' for the disease. We all know that memory loss, at varying degrees, is common among all human beings. In general, we tend to store procedural memory (memory of habits or procedures linked with a motor movement like self-feeding or tying a shoe) information longer than declarative memory (memory of facts such as anniversary dates, capital cities, famous people). Declarative memory information usually is the first to go yet patients who cannot remember their spouses names may be able to flawlessly demonstrate complicated knitting patterns or tie a fly for fishing that they have done repetitively for years.

In addition to retaining procedural-related information, we will be able to retain our long-term memory information much later in the disease process than information more recently acquired. The SLP working with this population should consider using strategies or methods of working with dementia patients that can tap into procedural memory skills as a way to help patients learn new habits (i.e., chin tuck for swallowing, word-finding strategies).

Early onset symptoms of memory loss may be subtle and inconsistent. Misplacing the car keys or forgetting faces and names can happen frequently and often are disregarded as a nuisance and a normal part of aging. In fact, it is not until later on in the disease process that most family members look back at the 'nagging' memory lapses and realize then that their loved one was presenting with dementia symptoms for many years before the memory loss became severe enough to impede normal functioning.

During this early phase of the dementia when memory loss is more of a nuisance would be the most optimal time to teach patient's new habits or patterns of behavior that they could use throughout the course of the dementia. Learning to write things down, using compensatory strategies such as journals or memory books, and systems of organization are very useful for this population in therapy. I usually tell my patients that learning to use compensatory strategies or systems for memory loss is similar to using a cane or walker to help with walking when the legs are weak . . . or using hearing aids when hearing acuity becomes impaired.

As the ability to retain new information deteriorates, the decline in normal independent functioning becomes more apparent. Forgetting to pay the gas bill, take medication, neglecting a pot of soup on the stove, and forgetting the way to the grocery store are examples of a level of memory impairment that can have a direct impact on a patient's quality of life and safety. Patients who begin to develop this level of memory impairment generally no longer can live at home without assistance or supervision. In this moderate stage of the dementia, the ability to utilize compensatory strategies may become more difficult as there also may be a progressive loss of fine or gross motor functions as well.

If the patient was used to writing notes for himself and has slowly lost the ability to write legibly, the clinician may need to find other ways to assist the patient with compensation (i.e., using large print labels or signs, using digital recorded memos).

As the dementia progresses into the later stages, and the ability to restore and recall information continues to deteriorate, the patient will begin to forget information once thought to be permanently engrained in the mind. He or she will be unable to retain the simple events of the day and/or the month, day, or year, even forgetting the names of children and grandchildren. Toward the later stages of the disease, patients may even demonstrate a deterioration of procedural memory patterns that impede independent self-care such as feeding, dressing, and toileting skills.

Although the inability to recall names or retain information for any period of time is a common characteristic of the late stages of dementia, it is important to note that patients often still can recall memories from long ago. They still may recall information from deep into their past as those types of memories are stored deeply in the brain. This is a good piece of information for the SLP to keep in mind when looking for 'stage appropriate' activities to engage in with patients during therapy. Using strategies to tap into spared long-term memory such as scrapbooks, photo albums, and old movies or music can be very helpful in the final stages of dementia.

Deterioration of Language Functioning

Although it is not considered a hallmark symptom of all dementias, it is very difficult to find a patient with dementia who does not suffer from some form of language dysfunction (aphasia). Depending on the area of the brain affected by the disease process, some patients will suffer from aphasic symptoms earlier in the disease and to a greater degree of severity than others. In addition, there will be different manifestations of the aphasia that may occur depending upon the type and severity of the disease. For instance, some patients may develop perseverations (word repetitions), while others may present with anomias (inability to find the word . . . not to be confused with the inability to articulate the word). As a clinician, it is important to assess language skills separate from memory skills. It can be easy to mistake a level of memory impairment during an examination when in reality, the patient suffered from an inability to produce verbal language.

Early on in the disease process, patients may have mild language deficits. Mostly described as the "tip of the tongue" syndrome where they feel as though the word will come to them at any moment. As these occasions are common to us all, the patient with dementia will exhibit them on a daily basis, often sighting increased frustration with communication. As a result, it is common for patients to begin to withdraw socially. Simple conversation can become frustrating and often embarrassing, leading to isolation. Higher functioning patients will begin to withdraw from social functions, avoiding activities that previously brought them a lot of satisfaction including church functions, book clubs, and volunteer activities. A patient who once enjoyed talking on the telephone may avoid the telephone altogether as it is now a source of tension and anxiety.

Written language and the act of writing may become difficult. This will directly impact and further compromise the patient's ability to handle personal finances, read and follow medication instructions on prescription bottles, or follow recipe instructions on food packages. It should be noted that the ability to process simple written words generally is spared much later into the disease process and can be a good tool for clinicians to tap into as a therapeutic intervention. We discuss this later in the book.

As the disease progresses, language ability may decline as well. Patients may begin to exhibit more "empty speech" eliminating nouns or pronouns from their vocabulary. Instead, using circumlocution or substituting words or phrases that will describe objects rather than naming them. The patient may say, "you know, that thing that you use to drink from" instead of saying the word "glass." Receptive language skills, or the ability to process and understand what is being said, may be affected as well. The deficits in receptive skills may greatly impact the patient's ability to retain information and should be taken into consideration during cognitive testing. If the patient does not understand the instructions given and is not able to process and encode the information accurately, it is not likely that the patient will be able to retrieve the information when needed as well.

Moving into the later stages, the ability to express basic wants and needs may become extremely difficult. The ability to let a caregiver know about hunger, thirst, pain, or bathroom needs may be difficult and create an enormous amount of anxiety and frustration. The patient's ability to use and comprehend nonverbal language still may be intact and should be assessed by the clinician. The use of communication boards and written signs/labels has been known to be very effective with patients who suffer from language deficits. It also should be noted that most patients who suffer from dementia still can retain the ability to interpret nonverbal cues such as facial expression, tone of voice, and body language.

Apraxia

The ability to execute motor functions, whether it is apraxia of speech or limb, affects many levels of daily functioning. The patient with dementia symptoms may have significant trouble following directions, both verbal and/or written. This would impact their ability to follow a new recipe or follow the exercises given by a physical therapist. It is most important for the clinician to be cognizant of this cognitive deficit, as it would impact the plan of care and the execution of certain therapeutic tasks. The dementia patient who suffers from apraxia may not be able to follow certain oral motor or physical exercises due to the motor planning impairment. Learning new sequences for dressing, brushing teeth, and swallowing compensatory strategies will have to be done via more creative modes, including more tactile cues and shorter learning sequences.

To be a little more descriptive of the speech/communication skills of the apraxic patient, Rosenbeck reports that patients with mild to moderately severe apraxia may grope inconsistently for the correct sound and may struggle awkwardly. They may be able to read and write much better than produce verbal output. They may be able to produce a multitude of spontaneous utterances but, once challenged to produce or repeat a specific word, struggle for accurate pronunciation if there is any output at all (Rosenbek, 1985).

The struggle for the clinician in diagnosing apraxia in the patient with dementia is the ability to get this patient to perform on cue during the examination. The clinician may need to take observations of different communication attempts and use that information to make a determination of apraxia. A method of doing this would be to engage the patient in general conversation about a specific topic (i.e., travel in the United States) and then have some specific words that the patient already had stated that should be repeated on command (i.e., Massachusetts, California, Mississippi). Words that are made up of multiple syllables can be especially difficult for the patient with apraxia (Rosenbek, 1985).

Agnosia

Persons with dementia may develop the inability to recognize familiar shapes, objects, persons, or sounds. Agnosia may impede a patient's ability to recognize the familiar faces of family members or even differentiate the sounds around them such as the telephone, the doorbell, or the television. Agnosia can be a cause for a great deal of confusion in the demented patient. The patient easily can become fearful if he or she is unable to recognize the people who are caring for them or understand that the loud sound they hear is the fire alarm and are unable to respond correctly. A person with agnosia may be able to name a familiar object or be able to identify the shape of an object but have no idea what the object is or how it is used. This deficit greatly impacts a patient's ability to function independently and safely in the home environment and generally will need the care and supervision of another individual.

Disturbances of Executive Functioning

Abstract thinking, planning and initiating, and sequencing and self-monitoring behaviors are all a part of executive functioning. The ability to regulate and prioritize tasks, organize thoughts and activities, as well as manage time efficiently all are affected by executive functioning. Deficits in executive functioning can relate to poor problem solving and judgment. These areas of thought, although considered a higher level of cognition, can have the greatest impact on the dementia patient's personal safety and ability to function independently. Deficits in the area of executive functioning are evident early on. The ability to effectively manage multiple activity of daily living tasks during a day is dependent upon executive functioning skills. Without this level of cognition, appointments would be missed as breakfast would last for hours. Prescriptions would not be filled and meals would not be purchased or prepared properly as the patient with dementia may not be able to plan appropriately to get to the store to purchase the right foods. Although executive functioning is considered a higher level of thought processes, it is paramount to safe, independent functioning. Patients with this level of deficit will not exist for long periods of time without outside intervention.

leading to other comorbidities including skin breakdown, malnutrition, dehydration, and aspiration pneumonia. The patient's physical deficits may have a direct relationship with cognitive decline as these deficits affect attention and focusing. As Parkinson's disease progresses, there is a greater likelihood that a reduction in cognitive processes will increase as well. Memory loss and other cognitive changes usually do not occur in Parkinson's disease until five to 25 years after the onset. It is more likely to occur in older individuals with more severe and longer duration of the disease and the presence of depression. Dementia occurs in Parkinson's dementia in more than 50% of individuals (Devere, 2011).

Frontal Temporal Dementia

This type of dementia is caused by disruption of the frontal and temporal lobes of the brain. There is no one specific abnormality associated with this type of disease. However, due to the area of the brain that is targeted, the behaviors of this disease are what sets it far apart from other dementias.

The frontal lobe of the brain is the gate keeper of our inhibitions. It is the filter for our social interactions and also plays a major role in our ability to pay attention, process, and problem solve. This type of dementia normally does not begin with memory loss. It begins with behavioral changes, often childlike and inappropriate. These individuals behave differently by saying things inappropriate, off color, or totally uncharacteristic to their normal personality. There may be a progessive inability to speak words and sentences but still understand them (Devere, 2011).

Other symptoms of this disease, also related to inhibitions, is excessive fluctuations of emotions rapidly moving from apathy to excessive happiness without apparent reason. These individuals also may demonstrate the inability to have adequate judgment when dealing with finances or even controlling apetite, often gaining excessive weight. Although there are no specific abnormalities associated with this disease, and this form of dementia still is quite rare, Pick's disease is the most common (Alzheimer's Association, 2012).

Normal Pressure Hydrocephalus (NPH)

This is one of the few dementias that can be altered or moderately reversed with intervention. Quick, accurate diagosis is very important with this type of dementia and can happen with astute observation of a unique set of symptoms. The first set of symptoms generally includes difficulty with walking and bladder control. Patients will have a sudden onset of a shuffeling gait or weakness leading to increased falls or near falls. Patients generally will complain of an increased sense of urgency and incontinence. "Usually after these physical developments progress, problems with memory, and other cognitive function begin to develop" (Devere, 2011).

The cause of NPH is a buildup of spinal fluid and brain pressure that can be treated successfully with a shunt tube placed in the spinal fluid cavity of the brain ventricles and drained through the neck, called a shunt (Devere, 2011).

Creutzfeldt-Jakob Disease (CJD)

According to the National Institute of Neurological Disorders and Stroke, CJD is an extremely rare disease, occuring in one out of one million people each year with approximately 200 cases identified each year. The cause is an abnormal clumping of proteins called prions in the brain, causing neuronal atrophy and death. The course of the disease is very rapid from the onset of symptoms, approximately six months to a year—which sets this dementia apart from the rest of the nonreversible dementias. The symptoms include a plethera of movement dysfunctions such as muscle stiffness, twitching, and jerkiness. Patients generally will suffer from increased occurrences of stumbling and falling. Some will suffer from blurred vision and hallucinations. All will present with increased confusion (National Institue of Neurological Disorders and Stroke, 2011).

Summary

Understanding the different manifestations and types of dementia can be valuable to the clinician in planning and implementing a plan of care. It is helpful to understand the characteristics that are common to the disease itself as a way for the clinician to be able to predict what assessments and tools might best fit the needs of the patient and be able to be well prepared prior to the appointment time. Even with all of this great knowledge, it still is important for the SLP to keep in mind that dementia is not the cause but a set of symptoms, and those symptoms may vary greatly from one individual to the next.

References

Alzheimer's Association. (2012). Alzheimer's disease facts and figures. *Alzheimer's & Dementia: The Journal of the Alzheimer's Association , 8*, 131–168.

Alzheimer's Disease Research. (2012). *A history of Alzheimer's disease.* Retrieved April 27, 2013, from Alzheimer's Association website at http://www.alz.org/research/science/alzheimers_research.asp

American Psychiatric Association. (2000). *Diagnostic and statistical manual of mental disorders (DSM-IV-TR)* (4th ed.). Arlington, VA: Author.

Devere, R. (2011). *Memory loss: Everything you want to know but forgot to ask.* Charleston, SC: CreateSpace.

National Institute of Neurological Disorders and StrokeInstitute of Health. (2011). *National Institute of Neurological Disorders and Stroke.* Retrieved April 27, 2013, from National Institutes of Health website at http://www.ninds.nih.gov/disorders/cjd/cjd.htm

Rosenbek, J. C. (1985). Treating apraxia of speech. In D. F. Johns & D. F. Johns (Eds.), *Clinical management of neurogenic communicative disorders* (p. 323). Boston, MA: College-Hill Press.

5

Physical Considerations: Look Beyond the Diagnosis

It is extremely rare to work with this population, or that of the elderly and aged in general, without having to deal with a handful of other physical and sometimes emotional/ behavioral deficits as well. This is what makes working with this population a little more complicated. The Alzheimer's Association reports that as of this year, AD is the sixth leading cause of death in the United States (Alzheimer's Association, 2012a). This may not be due to the development of the plaques and tangles in the brain but actually due to the numerous other effects and consequences on the body such as dysphagia or dehydration. The secondary physical and sometimes emotional symptoms that accompany the diagnoses of dementia are called comorbidities. It is rare for a patient with dementia to NOT exhibit comorbidities that further affect functioning, health, and often lead to the overall decline of the patient. For example, someone who has Parkinson's type dementia may develop difficulty with swallowing as a comorbidity. They then may develop aspiration pneumonia, which becomes difficult to treat and later leads to overall decline due to malnutrition and dehydration causing death. The diseases that cause dementia symptoms can affect so many other functions of the body, which have a direct impact on the overall health and well-being of the patient who has dementia. In this chapter, we will look a little deeper into the many comorbidities that are common to those who suffer from dementia.

Dysphagia

Dysphagia can be a result of behavioral, sensory, or motor problems (or a combination of these) and is common in individuals with neurologic disease and dementia. Although there are few studies of the incidence and prevalence of dysphagia in individuals with dementia, it is estimated that 45% of institutionalized dementia patients have dysphagia (Robbins & Easterling, 2008). Jeri Logemann reports that management of patients with dementia and dysphagia can be very complex. These patients may exhibit changes in behavior during meals, changes in physiology of swallow, and changes in cognitive or language function that affect their ability to understand or implement treatment strategies (Logemann, 2003).

The cause for the dysphagia will vary depending on the patient. Most swallow disorders occur in dementia patients due to a decrease in motor and sensory systems. For instance, patients may lose sensation in the oral cavity making it difficult to tell when food is adequately masticated. The patient may begin to demonstrate increased choking as food is not being chewed adequately. Patients may lose the ability to feel when the food has reached the point on the base of the tongue to trigger a swallow reflex, causing premature spilling of bolus before the airway can be sealed properly.

Other patients may suffer from impulsivity behaviors due to a dementia that interferes with the frontal lobe. Impulsive patients may eat very rapidly and put too much food in his or her mouth without knowing when to stop. Choking can occur easily with this patient as well as overeating. These patients may need to be closely monitored in the home or facilities where they have unlimited access to food as their lack of inhibition can cause them to go overboard in eating foods that are not good for them or cause harm if not prepared or chewed properly.

Decreased motor abilities that affect the oral cavity are a common occurrence in patients with dementia as well. Poor tongue control and decreased sensation will cause the patient to lose the ability to control the food in the mouth. Pocketing of food in the cheeks is very common in patients who have poor sensation as well as decreased self-perception. Pocketing of food can be very dangerous for the patient with dementia as it is difficult for the caregiver to tell there is residual food in the mouth. Patients who frequently pocket food are at risk for choking during meals as well as after, if they are allowed to recline directly after meals. The food that is pocketed then can travel down the throat without the patient initiating a swallow, causing choking or aspiration.

It is common for people with dementia to lose the ability to taste or smell certain foods. In fact, there is a real connection between smell and memory loss. The smell information travels from the nose to the medial temporal lobe (hippocampal region) of the brain. This is the area where short-term memory is stored. So disorders of this part of the brain can affect memory and smell, especially diseases such as Alzheimer' (Devere, 2011). This means that even though they do not recognize they have smell loss, individuals with Alzheimer's and Parkinson's dementia will likely develop an inability to recognize flavors, which can lead to weight loss, decreased appetite, and depression (Devere, 2011). Food that becomes bland tasting due to a decline in the ability to taste also can create a gag reflex in these patients. When eating becomes uncomfortable, or creates an unpleasant sensation either due to gagging or choking, patients may develop a subconscious aversion to oral intake. They may begin to associate intake as a negative situation and avoid eating altogether.

When these patients decrease their appetite, they will begin to lose weight. This can become a double-edged sword as the patient loses weight, their dentures or partials may become loose causing discomfort or sores on the gums or inner cheeks. Loose or ill-fitting dentition can make moving the food or liquid efficiently in the oral cavity difficult. Poor fitting dentures often are a cause of dysphagia and actually can interfere with the palate and the swallow mechanism, causing aspiration. This author actually has seen a patient with dementia swallow his own lower set of dentures during a meal!

Malnutrition

Malnutrition is poor nourishment resulting from improper diet or a defect in metabolism that prevents the body from using the energy properly. Symptoms of malnutrition can cause physical weakness and cause cognitive decline. Patients with dementia who are not getting appropriate nutrition, which can occur for a number of reasons, may exhibit a more rapid decline in cognition from lack of nutrients as opposed to a decline due to the disease causing the dementia. Malnutrition would be the prominent reason for weight loss in patients who have dementia. Alzheimer's disease is regularly connected with a signifi-cant and gradual loss of bodyweight; approximately 40% of Alzheimer's patients lose 4% bodyweight per year (Navratilova, Jarkovsky, Ceskova, Leonard, & Sabotka, 2007).

If malnutrition continues untreated, other symptoms may appear such as poor skin integrity, leaving the patient at further risk for wounds. This can become even more increas-ingly dangerous if the patient also becomes weakened and is forced to sit or lie down for most of his waking hours. The malnourished patient also may suffer from vision changes, fluid retention, and edema of the lower extremities. This occurs as the functioning of the internal organs such as the liver and kidneys are compromised due to lack of nutrition. Although malnutrition is common in patients who have more advanced dementia, very rarely are measures taken to provide artificial nutrition (i.e., tube feeding). A review of 77 studies conducted throughout 33 years found that tube feeding of advanced dementia patients offered absolutely no benefit and even caused some harm. The researchers concluded, "We identified no direct data to support tube feeding of demented patients with eating difficulties for any of the commonly cited indications" (Finucane, Christmas, & Travis, 1999).

Most often patients who develop more advanced symptoms of malnutrition are given to a hospice agency for care. Hospice caregivers are trained to identify and treat the signs and symptoms of malnutrition in patients with dementia.

Dehydration

As we get older, the thirst response becomes blunted and the ability for the mind to recog-nize the need for fluids diminishes. This of course worsens with the onset of dementia. Dehydration occurs when fluid intake is insufficient or output is excessive. Cognitive impairment has been associated with dehydration in older adults, thus making this a potentially reversible cause for some symptoms of dementia. Dehydration occurs more frequently in older adults who are frail and in those with diabetes, cancer, cardiac disease, or acute infections (such as urinary tract infections, upper respiratory infections, pneumonia, gastroenteritis, or skin infections) (Mentes, 2006). Due to some of the above factors (swallow problems, lack of awareness, etc.), it is easy for the demented patient to become dehydrated. There also are certain medications that can directly affect fluid balance in the body including diuretics, laxatives, and some psychotrophics. Polypharmacy also has been shown to heighten risk of dehydration. Studies have shown that there is a significant relationship between the use of four or more prescription medications and dehydration among elderly living in an institutional environment (Mentes, 2006).

Some of the indicators for dehydration include a darkening of the urine, dry skin, reduced saliva and drying of the tongue, sunken eyes, upper body weakness, and an increase in pulse rate. Historically, it has been commonplace to assess skin turgor for dehydration; it is not thought to be a reliable indicator in older adults because of changes in skin elasticity that occur with age (Mentes, 2006). Other common indicators of dehydration are a rapid onset of weakness and a leaning on one side or the other while sitting, standing, or walking. The clinician working with patients with dementia should make it a common practice to offer ample opportunities for hydration during treatment and make that part of the treatment plan with family and/or caregivers. The clinician should make it a priority to ensure that caregivers are adequately trained in the safest methods for the patient to get hydration, whether that be through a glass with a straw, a sippy cup with a lid, or a measured sip straw. Clinicians can teach caregivers some of the other ways to offer hydration with ice cream, popsicles, or fresh fruit such as citrus fruits or watermelon. Offering patients opportunities for hydration before, during, and after therapy sessions can make a huge difference in the patients health and hydration status. Clinicians should make a point to do this for all dementia patients.

Gum/Dental Disease

Dementia or the diseases that cause dementia do not cause gum or dental disease. It is the cognitive and physical effects of the disease and symptoms that cause a deterioration of the gums and dentition. The demented elderly need special care because they often suffer from extensive oral diseases causing tooth loss, gum disease, and oral fungus (thrush). The causes are general due to neglect as the hygiene routine in the demented is altered or neglected, and as the demented patient progresses into the later stages of the disease process, oral hygiene becomes increasingly challenging for caregivers due to uncooperative behaviors of the patient. The cognitive impact as well as the age-related changes in dentition is why more than 30% of facility-dwelling elderly in 1997 were edentulous (Helgeson, Smith, Johnsen, & Ebert, 2002). The SLP may see swallow deficits as a direct result of gum or dental disease including bleeding/sore gums, missing or abscessed teeth, or complications from neglected denture/partial hygiene. Providing oral care to patients that suffer from dementia can be very difficult. Some patients demonstrate fear and anxiety behaviors when approached to complete oral care. This may be due to confusion as to the purpose of the task or fear of pain and discomfort that occurs during oral care (particularly if there are sore gums and abscessed or rotting teeth!). Oral care should not be neglected. Even if the patient has dentures or partials, these need to be cleaned regularly on a daily basis to prevent infections. I have seen patients who had not removed their dentures for months and had to have them surgically removed as the food underneath had caused the dentures to fuse to the upper palate.

A major impact of systemic diseases on the oral health of older adults is caused by side effects of medications. With increasing age and associated chronic disease, the elderly are prescribed an ever expanding variety of medications. Adverse side effects of these medications may alter the integrity of the oral mucosa. Problems such as xerostomia (dry mouth), bleeding gums, tissue overgrowth, and hypersensitivity reactions may occur as a result of the drug therapy (Helgeson, Smith, Johnsen, & Ebert, 2002). Dental care in the Alzheimer's assisted living facilities and memory units is becoming more easily accessible with the increased availability of mobile dentist groups. By providing dental care at these facilities, a very large group of cognitively impaired individuals can gain access to primary rather than emergency dental care (Helgeson, Smith, Johnsen, & Ebert, 2002).

An important part of the SLP's plan of care should include training and education of caregivers and facility staff in proper and consistent oral care for the demented patient. Good oral care throughout the day can significantly reduce the risk for infections of the gum and respiratory system. The SLP also can partner with the occupational therapist working on skills for oral hygiene that the patient may be able to learn to do independently or with supervision from the caregiver. It also is helpful for the SLP to research dentists in the area that are skilled in treating patients who have dementia. There are some dentists that specially train their staff to work with these patients using calming techniques such as soothing music and soft lighting to keep patients quiet and calm during treatment. To help you locate dentists in your area that specialize in working with dementia, contact your local Alzheimer's Association chapter.

Infection

It is understood that as we age, we are more susceptible to infection and illness due to a natural breakdown of the different systems in the body that keep us healthy and stable. Systems such as the lymphatic system, respiratory system, and urinary system are only a few of the areas in the body that are responsible for filtering and cleansing the body to keep infection at bay. Natural aging causes these systems to deteriorate leaving the body open to illness and infection. Diseases or illness leading to dementia can further compromise these systems. Influencing factors leading to infection include exposure to infections in close community environments and medications that compromise the immune systems or stress current bodily systems. Medications such as sedatives and narcotics, anticholinergics, and gastric acid suppressants may affect the immune system. Malnutrition, which reduces cell immunity, is more common in the geriatric community. Functional impairments such as immobility, incontinence, and dysphagia can complicate aging and enhance susceptibility to infection (Strausbaugh, 2001).

When a normal, able-bodied individual, such as yourself, suffers from an infection (i.e., urinary tract infection), the symptoms can be difficult to identify. We can go throughout our normal day-to-day activities without noticing that we have an infection and usually do not have complaints until it becomes more serious. Most patients who suffer from dementia also often do not detect symptoms of infection. Just as it is difficult to identify the feelings of hunger or thirst, pain and discomfort often can be difficult to identify in individuals with dementia. The difference being that dementia patients can suffer through later, more serious stages of infection without being able to understand or communicate that they are sick. Furthermore, infections often can overrun systems in the body and have an overt affect on other normal uninfected parts of the body. For instance, a demented patient who is suffering from a urinary tract infection also may suffer from increased confusion as a result of the infection. Their walking and balance also may be affected with increased weakness causing an increase in the number of falls that are occurring. Oftentimes, it is difficult for us to tell whether or not these residual effects are from the infection or a precipitating factor such as dehydration.

The treating clinician needs to learn how to decipher these symptoms. Not that the SLP should take on the responsibility of identifying and diagnosing the comorbidities, but the SLP should pay attention to the signs and symptoms that the patient is exhibiting and report any peculiarities or changes in behavior to the physician or family members. Often changes due to infection will reverse themselves when an infection is identified properly and is diagnosed and treated with medication. The SLP can educate family and caregiver staff as to the specific individual behaviors that are exhibited by the patient when suffering from an infection. The ability for the caregiver to identify behaviors as being related to a specific infection will help prevent significant decline in overall functioning. Another intervention for the SLP is to work early on in teaching patients words or phrases that help identify pain or discomfort. Similarly, it is important for the SLP to teach/train caregivers to be able to identify other signs and symptoms of pain and discomfort when the patient cannot communicate verbally. Some of these signs may be increased anxious behaviors, rapid breathing, pacing, rocking back and forth, and so forth.

Gait Dysfunction

Gait dysfunction, or abnormality of gait, is when there is a deviation in normal walking. It further may be defined as slowed, aesthetically abnormal, or both and is not an inevitable consequence of aging but rather a reflection of the increased prevalence and severity of age-associated diseases (Alexander & Goldberg, 2005).

Research has shown us that the predominant cause of gait dysfunction in older adults is pain, followed by stroke and then visual loss (Alexander & Goldberg, 2005). For folks who have neurological impairment, the most common causes are related to cerebrovascular processes, sensory disorders, and Parkinson's disease (Alexander & Goldberg, 2005).

Gait dysfunction is likely to occur in patients who suffer from dementia as gait patterns are as much a complex cognitive process as is one requiring muscle strength and coordination. Unfortunately, falls are a common part of life for most patients who suffer from dementia, particularly in the later stages of the disease. Studies show annual fall incidences as high as 60% among people with dementia and as many as 400 falls per 100 persons with dementia (Shaw & Kenny, 1998). Although the SLP will not likely be responsible for improving gait dysfunction, falls can occur during therapy and the results of falling can greatly affect normal functioning. The SLP working on safety in the home setting may be called on to utilize cognitive-behavioral techniques to help patients learn to use modifications and assistive devices to reduce the risk of falls, like using a walker or cane. The SLP can work closely with the physical and occupational therapists to help establish appropriate goals and strategies creating an effective therapeutic environment to reduce falls and improve overall safety, despite the prevalence of gait dysfunction.

Heart Disease

According to the Centers for Disease Control, heart disease is the number one cause of death for people living in the United States. Furthermore, every 34 seconds, someone in the United States suffers from a heart attack (Centers for Disease Control and Prevention, 2012). We share this fact with you to illustrate that most of your elderly patients, whether they have dementia or not, are likely to suffer from heart disease. The list of predominant risk factors include being overweight, poor diet, and inactivity, which certainly can be commonplace among people with cognitive impairment, particularly in the later stages of the dementia. The SLP should be aware that a diagnosis of heart disease can be a contributing factor to symptoms of dementia. As you may recall from Chapter 4, vascular demetia is cuased by vascular changes, or changes in blood flow, in the brain. These changes, often referred to as mini strokes or TIAs (transient ischemic attacks), are the second leading cause of dementia in older adults. Vascular dementia can be the result of other changes in the brain from lack of blood flow, causing a depletion of vital nutrients and oxygen to the brain. Risks for vascular dementia include high blood pressure, high cholesterol, and smoking. Although the SLP will not be directly treating the heart disease, there always is an opportunity to educate family and caregivers on signs and symptoms of a heart attack (particularly if the patient is nonverbal) as well as good choices for better heart health through proper diet and exercise. This information may be a great benefit to the caregiver as well, who may be at greater risk for a heart attack due to the added stress of caregiving.

Sleep Disturbance

Sleep-wake disturbance is frequent in the demented elderly. Up to 50% of those with Alzheimer's dementia will have nocturnal restlessness and sleep-wake cycle reversal at some stage (Anderson, Hatfield, Kipps, Hastings, & Hodges, 2009). Sleep disturbance can compromise physical and cognitive functioning directly impacting performance of activities of daily living, not to mention goal-related performance in therapy. Patients who are sleep deprived are at greater risk for falls. These patients may suffer from an increase risk for dehydration and malnutrition as well due to being fatigued during the day and sleeping through meals. These patients may suffer from more stress-related illnesses, compromised immune systems, and increased confusion/disorientation related to fatigue or increased daytime sleeping. Patients who suffer from sleep disturbance also may be taking medications that are prescribed to help them sleep at night, which may be causing increased fatigue during the daytime hours as well. These medications can affect oral motor strength causing an increase in slurred speech or poor saliva control.

Although there is little that the SLP can do to directly impact sleep disturbance, it is good to be able to understand the consequences of sleep deprivation and how this can affect patients' overall attention and behavior in therapy, affecting outcomes. It is wise for the SLP to become aware of sleep patterns and make it a habit to check with caregivers prior to therapy as to whether the patient is well rested. It also is beneficial to make note of patterns of behavior that can be associated with fatigue. For example, I treated a patient with dementia who occasionally would suffer from falls. I noticed that the patient would fall on days where he did not sleep well the night before. I worked with the caregivers to enact extra safety precautions with this patient (i.e., supervision with ambulation at all times) on the days following a poor night's rest. We were successful at being able to reduce falls up to 75%.

Depression

The topic of depression in patients who have dementia almost deserves its own separate chapter. According to the CDC, 15 to 20% of adults older than age 65 in the United States have experienced depression. Seven million adults 65 and older are affected by depression, and people aged 65 years and older accounted for 16% of all suicide deaths in 2004 (Centers for Disease Control and Prevention, n.d.). These statistics do not factor in the diagnosis of dementia. It is estimated that 40% of the people who are diagnosed with Alzheimer's disease also suffer from depression (Alzheimer's Association, 2012b). The symptoms of depression alone can mirror the symptoms of dementia making diagnosis difficult at times. Apathy, loss of interest in activities or social events, and moodiness are all symptoms of both dementia and depression. Furthermore, the patient with dementia and depression is less likely to verbalize feelings of sadness or depression.

The clinician should be watchful for signs and symptoms of depression in patients who suffer from dementia. It is important to note if the patient has a history of depression or other mental illnesses, if there is a history of medical intervention for depression, and if the patient currently is taking any antidepressants or anti-anxiety medications.

According to the National Institute of Mental Health, the most common signs and symptoms of depression are: persistent sad, anxious, or "empty" feelings; feelings of hopelessness or pessimism; feelings of guilt, worthlessness, or helplessness; irritability; loss of interest in activities or hobbies once pleasurable; fatigue and decreased energy; difficulty concentrating, remembering details, and making decisions; insomnia, early morning wakefulness, or excessive sleeping; overeating or appetite loss; thoughts of suicide or suicide attempts; and aches or pains, headaches, cramps, or digestive problems that do not ease even with treatment (National Institute of Mental Health, 2012).

So what is the role of the SLP with depression? It is not our role to diagnose depression, but we should be keenly aware of symptoms, should they arise, and bring these observations immediately to the family, caregiver, and physician so that proper diagnosis and treatment can be implemented. Although I have no research data or evidence to prove that speech therapy can cure or lessen the effects of depression, I have noticed in my own personal practice that the one-on-one interaction with a SLP provides that close, personal interaction that sometimes is needed to clear away the gloom.

Summary

The list of physical considerations and comorbidities discussed in this chapter are only a few of many secondary symptoms that can develop in the dementia population. By understanding the comorbidities that often exist in dementia, the SLP will better be able to anticipate barriers that may arise during treatment and alter the plan of care accordingly to include goals that may address these issues. By looking at the comorbidities, the SLP is looking more holistically at the patient and maximizing overall care and outcomes.

References

Alexander, N. B., & Goldberg, A. (2005). Gait disorders: Search for multiple causes. *Cleveland Clinic Journal of Medicine, 72*(7), 586–600.

Alzheimer's Association. (2012a). Alzheimer's disease facts and figures. *Alzheimer's & Dementia: The Journal of the Alzheimer's Association, 8,* 131–168.

Alzheimer's Association. (2012b). *Depression and Alzheimer's.* Retrieved April 2, 2013, from http://www.alz.org

Anderson, K., Hatfield, C., Kipps, C., Hastings, M., & Hodges, J. (2009). Disrupted sleep and circadian patterns in frontotemporal dementia. *European Journal of Neurology, 16,* 317–323.

Centers for Disease Control and Prevention. (2012). *Heart disease fact sheet.* Retrieved April 2, 2013, from http://www.cdc.gov/dhdsp/data_statistics/fact_sheets/docs/fs_heart_disease.pdf

Centers for Disease Control and Prevention. (n.d.). *Healthy aging program.* Retrieved April 2, 2013, from http://www.cdc.gov/aging/pdf/CIB_mental_health.pdf

Devere, R. (2011). *Memory loss: Everything you want to know but forgot to ask.* Charleston, SC: CreateSpace.

Finucane, T., Christmas, C., & Travis, K. (1999). Tube feeding in patients with advanced dementia: A review of the evidence. *Journal of the American Medical Association,* 1365–1370.

Helgeson, M. J., Smith, B. J., Johnsen, M., & Ebert, C. (2002). Dental considerations for the frail elderly. *Special Care in Dentistry, 22,* 40–55.

Logemann, J. A. (2003, February 18). Dysphagia and dementia: The challenge of dual diagnosis. *ASHA Leader.* Retrieved April 5, 2013, from http://www.asha.org/Publications/leader/2003/030218/030218g.htm

Mentes, J. (2006). Oral hydration in older adults. *American Journal of Nursing,* 40–49.

National Institute of Mental Health. (2012). *Depression.* Retrieved April 5, 2013, from http://www.nimh.nih.gov/health/publica tions/depression/index.shtml

Navratilova, M., Jarkovsky, J., Ceskova, E., Leonard, B., & Sabotka, L. (2007). Alzheimer disease: Malnutrition and nutritional support. *Clinical and Experimental Pharmocology and Physiology,* 11–13.

Robbins, E., & Easterling, C. (2008). *Dementia and dysphagia.* Retrieved April 30, 2013, from http://www.ncbi.nlm.nih.gov

Shaw, F., & Kenny, R. (1998). Can falls in patients with dementia be prevented? *Age and Aging, 27*(1), 7–9.

Strausbaugh, L. J. (2001). Emerging health care-associated infections in the geriatric population. *Emerging Infectious Diseases, 7*(2), 268–271.

PART

Effective Therapeutic Interventions

Part II of this book is divided into four chapters. Chapter 6 focuses on "Dementia Staging." It addresses the current staging tools used for dementia and how each stage relates to the daily functioning, communication needs, and behaviors of the patient with dementia. Our hope is that this information can assist the SLP in providing current education to the professionals and caregivers working with the patient with dementia. Chapter 7 focuses on how to effectively evaluate the patient with dementia, from the referral process to screenings to chart reviews, and a discussion of both formal and functional evaluation processes for this population. Chapter 8 looks at setting goals for persons with dementia. Detailed descriptions of the anatomy of a well-written and reimbursable goal are shared, along with examples of goals focused on the domains of communication, intake, and cognition. Finally, Chapter 9 looks at the current treatment trends for the SLP or other rehabilitation professional working with the dementia population. Evidenced-based practice is the focus of this chapter, along with a detailed case study of how to utilize the approaches discussed in the chapter in patient treatment.

CHAPTER

6

Dementia Staging

The practice of evaluating and treating patients who suffer from dementia is not an exact science. It is not uncommon during my practice for family members to ask me to tell them how long their loved one will live, or "how long will it be before they don't know who I am?" It is devastating to know that your loved one suffers from a disease that ultimately will steal their memory and most all bodily control. Just as horrifying is knowing that your loved one may have to suffer emotional and physical discomfort through the progression of the disease. With all of the uncertainty that comes with a diagnosis of dementia, what is certain is that there is no way to predict the future. Although we are better at developing ways to diagnose and treat dementia, the progression of the disease and the impact that the symptoms have on daily functioning is hard to predict. The factors of environment, overall health and comorbid conditions, as well as the available care and competence of caregivers all can have an impact on the progression of dementia. This chapter will provide some information regarding some of the diagnostic tools available to clinicians to help assess and plan for treatment and future care of the dementia patient.

Throughout the years, scientists have observed similar characteristics of behaviors in people who suffer from dementia. It also has been observed that people diagnosed with dementia take a somewhat similar downward trajectory with the decline of levels of functioning. Several tools have been developed to help healthcare professionals identify the varying stages of functioning and decline. For a SLP, the use of these staging tools in conjunction with the usual battery of diagnostic tests can be beneficial in developing a treatment plan as well as providing education and support to family and caregivers. Knowledge and use of these tools can assist the clinician in understanding behavior characteristics that can be expected when greeting the patient for the initial evaluation as well as understanding that unusual new behaviors may be an indication into the progression of the dementia to another level. The SLP as part of a treatment team that includes the physical therapist (PT), occupational therapist (OT), nurse, social worker, caregiver, and physician can use staging tools to look at the patient on the same level, use the same vocabulary and terminology, as well as have a mutual understanding as to the direction the patient is headed.

Staging tools are not predictors of how a patient will progress with regard to a time line. As mentioned previously, there are so many other factors that influence the progression of the disease. It is impossible to predict when one will move from one stage to the next. It also is possible that one patient may progress more rapidly than others, often skipping a stage or two along the way. It is rare that a patient moves in the opposite direction, moving backward through the staging system. However, it is possible that with the elimination of certain factors that cause temporary cognitive impairment or "reversible dementia," patients can show an improvement in behaviors or functions that may have him or her improve to a previous level.

For years, the medical community has referred to a staging system published by The American Psychiatric Association's *Diagnostic and Statistical Manual of Mental Disorders*, Third Edition (DSM-III), which recognized a staging system consisting of three stages of progression (Reisberg et al., 2011).

Early Stage

This stage often is overlooked and seen as a normal part of aging. The evidence of symptoms are subtle and may include difficulty with language and word finding. There may be problems with short-term memory, and patients may repeat themselves. There also may be frequent but not constant disorientation to time or place, as well as trouble making decisions and executing actions. Accompanied with these changes often is a subtle change in mood with depressive symptoms and lack of interest in hobbies and interests or socialization. People in this stage also may occasionally act out of character with anger or aggression at unpredictable times.

The SLP may or may not interact with these individuals in therapy. It is rare that patients are able to detect these symptoms on their own and seek the assistance of the SLP independently. It is not uncommon for patients to demonstrate complete denial of their own cognitive deficits well into the latter part of this early stage. This denial of deficit creates a significant barrier to treatment for the therapist as it is difficult to "fix" something unless one knows that it is "broken." Conversely, patients may have an awareness that something is not right with their mentation and develop a defensive attitude toward anyone who offers to assist. This frequently puts the SLP in an uncomfortable situation. Oftentimes, the SLP also will be working with family members in assisting them in how to deal with their loved one's journey into dementia. Once the SLP is able to work through the barrier of denial, the most common emphasis of therapy during this stage is teaching compensatory strategies. Teaching patients to get used to using assistive devices for memory during this stage will help them to establish good habits later on in the disease process, keeping them functional and independent for as long as possible.

Middle Stage

As the disease progresses, deficits become more evident and limitations become clearer and more prominent affecting day-to-day functioning. People at this stage may demonstrate increased forgetfulness of recent events or the names of close family or friends. There is an increase in problems managing household tasks such as cooking, cleaning, and maintenance. Personal hygiene may become difficult or neglected due to forgetfulness. There is an increased dependence on family members or caregivers for help in the home. There also may be an increase in personal accidents with falls becoming more common due to poor judgment, visual perception, and even incontinence. Speech and language deficits may become more prominent and behaviors such as repetitive questioning, calling out, acting out, and getting lost in once familiar surroundings is more common.

This is where the SLP needs to get more creative in treating these patients as the real world and the ability to reason rapidly begin to slip away. SLPs may be teaming up with the OTs and PTs on goals related to functional activities of daily living and safety. Priorities for therapy evolve from being a focus on compensatory strategies for the patient for complete independence, to strategies and cueing methods that the caregiver can employ to help the patient function at their highest level under supervision. Another focus for the SLP will be finding ways to help alter and eliminate behaviors such as repetitive questioning and wandering. Patients at these levels still may have spared ability to read labels and follow simple cuing systems to keep them safe.

Late Stage

The characteristics of late stage dementia are severe enough to necessitate complete dependence on caregivers for all basic needs. Persons at this stage may need help to be fed meals, be incapable of communicating or understanding what is being said to them, have trouble walking, swallowing, toileting, or initiating any movements at all, and may be confined to a wheelchair. People at this stage may display inappropriate and unpredictable behavior.

The focus for the SLP now turns to finding ways to help the patient remain comfortable, healthy, and safe. Generally, there is an emphasis on basic life functioning skills such as eating food, swallowing liquids and medications, and expressing basic needs such as hunger, thirst, or pain. Treatment time with patients in these later stages of the disease process tends to be shorter than when working with patients in the earlier stages. A big emphasis in treatment is caregiver education and training—not only in how to carry through with the strategies developed in therapy but also in helping caregivers understand how strategies may need to be modified and adapted as the disease progresses to the end.

Functional Stages in Normal Human Development and Alzheimer's Disease (Table 6–2)

Dr. Reisberg also developed an effective staging tool that links a patient's Alzheimer's stage with a person's developmental age and acquired and lost abilities. This tool might be useful in determining appropriate materials and activities to use during therapy and to recommend to family and caregivers.

Axial and Multiaxial Staging

Axial and multiaxial staging takes dementia staging another step further by combining assessment tools that look at a number of different individual assessment areas such as concentration, recent memory, orientation, long-term memory, short-term memory, and so forth, along with the global deterioration scale to get a more detailed depiction of the stage of dementia. As these tools are for more advanced diagnostic needs, such as differential diagnosis of dementing disorders, we will not go into depth with explanation of these tools. These assessment techniques and staging methods are more time consuming for the clinician and more difficult to use as an education tool for family members and caregivers. The most commonly used axial and multiaxial tools are written by Barry Reisberg,

Table 6–2. Functional Stages in Normal Human Development and Alzheimer's Disease

Approximate Age	Acquired Abilities	Lost Abilities	Alzheimer's Stage
12+ years	Hold a job	Hold a job	3—incipient
8–12 years	Handle simple finances	Handle simple finances	4—mild
5–7 years	Select proper clothing	Select proper clothing	5—moderate
5 years	Put on clothes unaided	Put on clothes unaided	6—moderately severe
4 years	Shower unaided	Shower unaided	
4 years	Toilet unaided	Toilet unaided	
3–4½ years	Control urine	Control urine	
2–3 years	Control bowels	Control bowels	
15 months	Speak 5–6 words	Speak 5–6 words	7—severe
1 year	Speak 1 word	Speak 1 word	
1 years	Walk	Walk	
6–10 month	Sit up	Sit up	
2–4 months	Smile	Smile	
1–3 months	Hold up head	Hold up head	

Copyright © 1984 by Barry Reisberg, M.D. Reproduced with permission.

entitled the Brief Cognitive Rating Scale (BCRS) published in 1982, and the Functional Assessment and Staging Tool (FAST) published in 1984 (Reisberg, 1984; National Institutes of Health, n.d.). Both tools still are available for use today by Geriatric Resources Inc.

Summary

Staging tools are a wonderful diagnostic resource and education tool for the clinician and the entire team working with the patient with dementia. Even when the patient's skill levels and deficits fluctuate from day to day, which frequently happens because of comorbidities like fatigue and medication interaction, the clinician can step back and take a good look at a patient's overall functioning to place them in a specific stage of dementia. The ability to find a common ground among the entire healthcare team, family members, and caregivers using the various staging tools available allows for a more cohesive plan of approach to the care of these patients.

References

Alzheimer's Research Center. *New diagnostic criteria and guidelines for Alzheimer's disease.* Retrieved April 2011, from http://www.alz.org/research/diagnostic_criteria

National Institutes of Health. (n.d.). *National Institute on Aging.* Retrieved April 10, 2013, from http://www.nia.nih.gov/alzheimers

Reisberg, B. (1984). *The functional assessment staging test of dementia.* Radium Springs, NM: Geriatric Resources.

Reisberg, B. (1988). Functional Assessment Staging (FAST). *Psychopharmacology Bulletin, 24,* 653–659.

Reisberg, B., Ferris, S., DeLeon, M., & Crook, T. (1982). The global deterioration scale for assessment of primary degenerative dementia. *American Journal of Psychiatry, 139,* 1136–1139.

Reisberg, B., Imran, J. A., Khan, S., Monteiro, I., Torossian, C., Ferris, S., . . . Wegiel, J. (2011). Staging dementia. *Principles and Practice of Geriatric Psychiatry, 3,* 162–168.

7

Evaluation Tools and Techniques

The evaluation process is a crucial step for any therapist when beginning to work with a patient. There are many variables involved in this process, beyond just choosing an appropriate standardized test, particularly when evaluating a patient with dementia. Variables such as the patient's current state of health, additional services the patient is receiving, the environment available for testing, and the functional needs of the patient, their family, and/or facility/paid staff are all important considerations for beginning the evaluation process for a patient with dementia. In this chapter, we will focus not only on how to choose appropriate testing materials but also how to factor in these additional variables to develop an effective and functional plan of care for our dementia patients.

Referrals

If you are working in a skilled nursing, outpatient, or home care setting, the referral from the patient's physician for a speech therapy evaluation may only end up on your desk, waiting expectantly for you to complete it. In this case, you already have the "green light" to move forward and see this patient. These referrals may have been generated from the patient's physician or discharge planner from the hospital and are likely related to other conditions the patient may be experiencing, such as swallowing difficulty. However, in other cases, the SLP may have to assist in the referral being obtained from the physician. This sometimes occurs when the patient is being seen by other disciplines such as skilled nursing or physical or occupational therapy, and these professionals are noticing that the patient is having a difficult time responding to their treatment due to their memory difficulties. These professionals then may suggest to the patient themselves, their family, or facility staff that speech therapy may benefit the patient. Many times, the physician is agreeable to providing an initial order for an evaluation and then will require follow up from the SLP regarding the patient's response to treatment. Sometimes, however, the physician may be less agreeable to this and may hold the mistaken belief that patients with dementia cannot benefit from skilled rehabilitation treatment due to their memory and/or behavioral deficits. It then becomes the job of the SLP to educate the physician on our scope of practice with dementia, and how we can provide instruction that can benefit not only the patient but also the patient's caregivers on how to compensate for the patient's progressive difficulties with speech, language, swallowing, and behavior. Information provided in this manual can assist the SLP in educating referral sources as to how speech therapy can benefit patients with dementia. We refer you to the Appendix for worksheets that can be used to assist in this process.

Insurance providers are another piece of the referral/evaluation puzzle. Physicians may provide the order for speech evaluation and therapy, but often the patient's insurance company may have other ideas about authorizing evaluation and treatment. The physician order always takes priority over insurance authorization, but the patient's and/or the patient's power of attorney **must be notified** by you at the initiation of service that they may be responsible for payment if their insurance decides not to authorize services. Again, you as the speech pathologist may have to take the role of educator for the insurance company regarding scope of practice for speech pathology, focus of evaluation and treatment, and caregiver education. Position statements and technical reports created by the American Speech-Language-Hearing Association (ASHA) are important documents to have at your fingertips to define the SLP's scope of practice related to dementia. "The Roles Speech-Language Pathologists Working With Individuals With Dementia-Based Communication Disorders: Technical Report and Position Statement" (ASHA, 2005a, 2005b) both can be accessed through the ASHA website and is listed in the "References" at the end of this chapter. We continue to address the important area of physician, payor source, and caregiver education throughout this manual.

There also may be times when the speech pathologist is looking to generate referrals in order to build a stronger caseload. The best and most efficient way to accomplish this is to provide education to the referral sources, including physicians and other professional disciplines, including nurses, physical and occupational therapists, social workers, discharge planners, and caregiving staff. When these professionals are better informed as to how speech pathologists can assist patients with dementia and provide ongoing support, education, and instruction to the patients' care, they are more likely to make a referral for service. Many times, professionals and families are unaware of what speech therapists do beyond "helping people talk better" or "helping people eat better." It is our job to be our own advocates and educate the broad range of services we can provide to patients, including those with dementia. Professionals and families also may believe that patients no longer can learn or recall information and would be unable to participate in treatment. Again, information in this manual should be used to educate referral sources as to how learning and memory works, and how we as SLPs can assist both the patient and their caregivers through skilled instruction. We have created a "Referral Checklist" that can be used to help identify patients who may benefit from speech therapy services. It is listed as Figure 7–1.

Referral Checklist for Dementia

Please read the following list of common difficulties related to dementia and check any that apply to your patient. These concerns may warrant a referral for a full speech therapy evaluation. Please return and direct any questions to:

_____

Speech-Language Pathologist; Office #; Telephone #

_____

Patient Name/Initials; Room Number

Does the patient?

_____ Seem "more forgetful" lately? For example, forgetting recent events or the names of important people in their life.

_____ Appear to have more trouble completing daily routines or need more assistance in complete common activities?

_____ Forget the names of common objects in their living environment or tends to "search for words" when speaking?

_____ Tend to ask the same questions repeatedly throughout the day and/or not recall asking the question or recall the answer to their question?

_____ Seem to be misplacing common items more frequently and are unable to retrace their steps to find items?

_____ Have trouble with regularly knowing the date, time, or season, or knowing where they are?

_____ Withdraw from social activities or activities they once enjoyed participating in?

_____ Exhibit behaviors that are out of character, such as aggression, confusion, combativeness, wandering, and so forth?

_____ Been exhibiting difficulties with judgment or decision making related to their own safety, finances, and so forth?

_____ Seem more confused with visual images, such as difficulty reading or not recognizing their image in a mirror?

Figure 7–1. Referral checklist for dementia.

Screening

Screening often may be part of the evaluation process when working with patients with dementia. This typically occurs in a facility setting, such as a skilled nursing facility, and may be part of the facility's ongoing assessment of their patients needs. Screening is a non-billable service and generally consists of a patient's chart review, brief interviews with facility staff and/or the patient's family, and a brief observation of the patient in his/her environment. Many times, screenings are performed when a patient is initially admitted to a facility but also can be conducted on staff or family recommendation, or to coincide with the facility's care plan schedule. It is important to check a facility's policy related to screening for rehabilitation and follow it accordingly. In general, however, screening can lead to the identification of patient needs that may be assisted and/or improved through skilled speech therapy services. This information can be used as justification to request a referral from the patient's physician for a full speech therapy evaluation. There are many commercially available screening measures available today. We will limit our discussion here to a few of the most current and commonly used in the field. Table 7–1 below summarizes the Mini-Mental State Examination (MMSE; Folstein, Folstein, & McHugh, 1975), the Saint Louis University Mental Status Examination (SLUMS; Tariq & Morley, 2006), the Clock Drawing Test (numerous versions), the Spaced Retrieval Screen (Brush & Camp, 1998), and the Montreal Cognitive Assessment (MoCA; Nasreddine, et al., 2005). We advise that any screening measure recommended for use with the dementia population be fully reviewed first by the SLP and chosen based on the needs of the patient and the information you wish to glean from it.

Evaluation Considerations

Prior to administering a standardized test with a dementia patient, it is important to consider a number of variables that may impact the patient's performance. In their 2005 Technical Report, ASHA highlights the importance of assessing the patient's sensory abilities. "Hearing loss is particularly common among older adults in long-term care settings (Hull, 1995; Voeks, Gallagher, Langer, & Drinka, 1990), as is visual impairment" (ASHA, 2005b). Prior to evaluating the patient, you will want to determine what his/her sensory deficits are and be sure to accommodate for these during testing. Making sure the patient has and is wearing properly working hearing aids if needed, has ear canals that are free of impacted wax, and is wearing glasses if prescribed are important elements of the patient performing well during the assessment process. If the patient hears better on one side versus another, you will want to work on that side to allow them to perform to their highest potential. If the patient has visual deficits, you may need to adapt and modify your materials to be in larger, easier-to-read print. We address print size and visual accommodations further in Chapter 9.

It also is important to make sure the assessment environment is conducive to allow the patient to perform at the highest level possible. If sitting at a table for the evaluation,

Table 7–1. Common Screening Measures Used With Dementia

Screening Measure	Areas Assessed	Administration Time	Scoring
Mini Mental State Examination (MMSE; Folstein, Folstein, & McHugh, 1975)	• Assesses global cognitive function, with items assessing orientation, word recall, attention and calculation, language abilities, and visuospatial ability • Widely used	Takes approximately 10 minutes to administer	Scores range from 0–30; scores below 25 indicate some impairment; scores between 11–24 indicate mild to moderate dementia; scores less than 10 indicate severe impairment
Saint Louis University Mental Status Examination (SLUMS; Tariq & Morley, 2006)	• Assesses orientation, short-term memory, calculations, naming of animals, clock drawing, and recognition of geometric figures • Nonproprietary; free to download and use	Takes approximately 7 minutes to administer	Scores range from 0–30 with scores of 27–30 considered normal in a person with a high school education; scores between 21–26 suggest mild neurocognitive disorder; and scores between 0–20 indicate dementia
The Clock Drawing Test (numerous versions)	• Assesses general cognitive and adaptive functioning such as memory, information processing, executive functioning, and vision • Results of test have been studied and compared to MMSE performance	Administration time can be anywhere from 1–5 minutes	Scoring and interpretations vary
Spaced Retrieval Screen (Brush & Camp, 1998)	• Assesses patient's ability to recall information over spaced intervals of time • Indicates if patient may benefit from use of spaced retrieval technique to recall information	Administration time 1–3 minutes	Scoring is pass or fail based on performance
The Montreal Cognitive Assessment (MoCA; Nasreddine et al., 2005)	• Assesses short-term memory recall, visuospatial abilities, executive function, attention, concentration, working memory, language, and orientation • Useful for early detection of mild cognitive impairment (MCI) and early Alzheimer's disease • Nonproprietary; free to download and use	Approximately 10 minutes to administer	Scores range from 0–30 with a score of 26 or above considered "normal"

try to keep the tabletop as clear as possible. Try to keep all testing materials off of the table on the floor next to you and present materials only when needed. Not only is seeing a pile of paperwork or testing booklets overwhelming and scary to the patient, it also can cause the patient to become distracted. Choosing a quiet area with adequate lighting and minimal distractions is recommended but may not always be possible. At times, the SLP may have to evaluate in the patient's facility room, which may or may not be private, in the patient's home, which may have other family members or additional distractions present, or in a facility dining area, especially if the patient is being evaluated for swallowing difficulties. These again are not the optimum assessment environments but can be considered functional and representative of where the patient typically spends their day and how they function within in it, which will provide you with important information not only about the patient's abilities and deficits but also how likely to proceed with treatment.

The patient's culture, native language, and religious beliefs also should be considered prior to assessing the patient. Ask family and/or available staff about any particular considerations that should be kept in mind regarding these areas when working with the patient, and make a note on your evaluation materials so that you are able to remember them. It also is recommended to find out what time of day is best to see the patient. Some patients with dementia may demonstrate "sundowning" characteristics. The Mayo Clinic defines sundowning as "a state of confusion at the end of the day and into the night. Sundowning isn't a disease, but a symptom that often occurs in people with dementia, such as Alzheimer's disease. The cause isn't known." (Mayo Clinic, 2011). If the patient demonstrates sundowning behavior, it may be best to see the patient earlier in the day to circumvent this deficit.

Having a thorough knowledge of the patient's current state of overall health is crucial in structuring the evaluation. Prior to seeing the patient, you will want to make every effort to know the patient's full list of diagnoses, their medications and time of day they are administered, and any additional disciplines or appointments the patient may have to work with or attend. All of these areas will impact the patient's overall performance during evaluation. Here are a few examples of these considerations.

- If a patient has some medications administered directly after lunch, some of which can cause drowsiness, you may want to time your evaluation to be prior to lunch to achieve a better estimate of the patient's abilities.

- If a patient also is being seen by physical and occupational therapists, you will want to plan your evaluation around those times so that the patient is not overly fatigued when being tested.

- If the patient attends dialysis on Tuesdays and Thursdays, you will want to schedule your evaluation on Monday, Wednesday, or Friday so that they are feeling their best when you see them.

- If the patient loves to play BINGO and the facility has it scheduled at 2 PM each day, you will want to see this patient before or after the activity occurs. This will help you start off "on the right foot" with the patient and not force the patient to miss something they enjoy doing to participate in testing.

Sometimes, no matter how hard you to try to accommodate for the patient's schedule and needs, you may need to evaluate the patient at a "less than optimal" time. When this occurs, it is just important to note that the patient's performance may have been impacted by additional factors, and the assessment results may not be a true depiction of the patient's abilities. When this occurs, the need to conduct ongoing assessment of the patient during treatment becomes a greater priority.

Chart Review and Case History

A patient with dementia living in a facility setting typically has a medical record or chart that should be thoroughly reviewed by the speech pathologist prior to evaluating the patient. It is important to schedule time prior to assessing the patient with the chart in order to better understand that patient's health history, medications, and family and psycho-social history. By conducting a thorough chart review, the SLP can obtain a better idea of who the patient is and what other issues, both health and non-health related, the patient is dealing with at the time. As stated above, this information can inform the SLP's decisions regarding day and time to best schedule the patient's evaluation and other accommodations that may need to be made to the testing materials or the testing environment. When reviewing the patient's chart, it also is recommended to gather information regarding the patient's former occupation, hobbies, names of family members, and so on, as this information can be used to help build an initial rapport with the patient at evaluation and can be used to create meaningful treatment materials to address the patient's goals.

In settings outside of facilities, such as home health care, the SLP may have limited access to a thorough case history of the patient. In these cases, it is recommended that the SLP try to gather information from other disciplines who already may be working with the client, such as the nurse or physical therapist, or to ask some initial case history questions over the phone when calling to schedule the evaluation. The more information you have prior to seeing the patient, the better and more individualized the evaluation will be. Below are a few examples of quick case history questions that can be asked of other disciplines or to the patient's family prior to the evaluation visit.

- What is the best time of day to visit the patient?
- Is the patient aware of their memory deficit?
- Is the patient facing multiple health issues at this time?
- What did the patient do for a living?
- What does the patient enjoy doing now (hobbies, interests, etc.)?
- What does the family member, caregiving staff, or other home health providers feel are areas that speech therapy might assist with?

When the time comes to actually meet with the patient, you also will want to be prepared to ask them some questions to get a sense of how they are functioning and how they feel about their memory. This is particularly important with patients in the early stages of dementia, as they can answer these questions more directly. If the patient you are evaluating is in the moderate-to-late stages of dementia, you will likely want to direct your questions to the patient's family and/or caregivers, as they can likely provide more reliable responses. There are assessments available, such as the Quality of Life-AD (QOL-AD; Logsdon, Gibbons, McCurry, & Teri, 1999), which can be used to interview both the patient and the patient's caregivers regarding their perception of their quality of life, including areas of physical health, memory, and life as a whole.

When meeting with the patient for the first time, be prepared to explain your role as a speech therapist and what you can do to help them. Many times, the patients may be in denial about their memory issues, their family may have requested the evaluation, or the patient and family may be unaware of the speech therapist's role in treating cognitive issues. This should all be explained before any formal testing begins. You may need to "tread lightly" here as you tell the patient/family why you are meeting with them. We have found that the best approach is to explain that you are there to help make their life a bit easier, whether that is through remembering things better or learning some new ways to do things, and that you want them to be involved in the process to make your visits/sessions as meaningful as possible and a good use of their time.

There are many commercially available case history forms available for use during the evaluation process. Use the one provided by your employer or facility or one that you feel the most comfortable in using. In addition to the common case history questions, we recommended including the following questions in your initial patient and/or caregiver interview.

- Tell me how you feel about your memory. Are you having any trouble remembering certain things throughout the day? Tell me about them.
- If you could wave a magic wand and remember anything a little better, what would you want to remember?
- What are some ways you try to remember better or keep track of things? I usually make lists and use a calendar. What do you do? Are these things working for you right now?
- Are there any social situations or activities that you once enjoyed that you find more difficult to participate in now? Tell me about those. What makes these situations difficult for you?
- Tell me about how you spend your day? What do you like to do? What are some things you wish you still could do or do a little more easily?
- Do you have any favorite T.V. shows? If you enjoy reading, what do you like to read?
- For the caregiver, what are some things you wish your loved one could remember better? What are your biggest concerns or priorities for me to address with your loved one in treatment? Caregivers also may be able to provide answers to some of the personal interest/hobby questions if the patient is unable to tell you directly.

Obtaining the answers to these questions will help to provide you with information regarding how the patient feels about their memory and their abilities. Knowing details such as favorite T.V. shows and reading material can help you to develop more meaningful treatment materials and activities. Adding this information to your evaluation results will help in creating more individualized treatment for your patients.

Selected Formal Tests for Evaluating Dementia

Depending on the setting in which you work, the time allotted for evaluation may vary. Selecting an appropriate test for formally evaluating a patient with dementia should include knowing the length of time you have available to see the patient, related to both patient health status and possible fatigue, and the amount of time that is billable for reimbursement. Here we list a few formal assessments that are commercially available for use by the SLP for evaluation of the dementia patient.

- Arizona Battery for Communication Disorders of Dementia (ABCD; Bayles & Tomoeda, 1993)
  - For ages 15 and older (with TBI)
  - Testing time 45 to 90 minutes
  - Can be administered individually or in a group
  - Includes 14 subtests that can be given separately or collectively
  - Assesses linguistic expression, linguistic comprehension, verbal episodic memory, visuospatial construction, and mental status.
- Ross Information Processing Assessment-Geriatric, Second Edition (RIPA G-2; Ross-Swain & Fogle, 2011)
  - For ages 55 years and older
  - Testing time 25 to 35 minutes
  - Administered individually
  - Includes seven subtests that can be combined to form an overall Information Processing Index
  - Assesses areas such as immediate memory, spatial orientation, categorical vocabulary, and listening comprehension.
- Repeatable Battery for the Assessment of Neuropsychological Status (RBANS; Randolph, 1998)
  - For ages 20 to 89 years
  - Administration time 30 minutes
  - Assesses several different areas of cognitive functioning
  - Can be used as a screening tool and/or to track recovery during rehabilitation and to track progression of degenerative diseases, like dementia.

In 2007, Mahendra and Apple published in *The ASHA Leader* a user-friendly table to assist the SLP in the decision-making process for choosing an assessment with dementia. This information can be accessed at the following website: http://www.asha.org/uploaded Files/Publications/leader/2007/071127/f071127a3.pdf (Mahendra & Apple, 2007).

Functional Evaluation

Along with formal assessment, it is critical to evaluate the functional needs of the patient at evaluation. This means conducting "informal assessment" of the patient within their environment. Functional or informal assessment translates to gathering information on the patient's functional skills in a nonstandardized manner. Using this information in conjunction with the results of the patient's performance on standardized measures helps to paint a clearer picture of the patient and can provide the clinician with important information, such as level and type of cueing needed by the patient to achieve success. Below are some examples of informal, functional assessment tasks that can be included in the patient evaluation. These informal assessments may at first be viewed as perhaps "tricking" or being dishonest with the patient, but we have found that many times asking these questions or setting up scenarios like these help the patient to not feel as though they are being tested, and because some of them require the therapist to seem disorganized or forgetful, it can make the patient feel more at ease about their own memory issues.

- Informal Memory/Orientation Assessment Examples:
  - Telling the patient a brief story about yourself (your name, where you grew up, information about your family or your hobbies), then asking the patient to summarize the information back to you or ask specific questions regarding the story.
  - Filling out your assessment paperwork in front of the patient and asking questions, such as, "Can you tell me your room number or address so that I can have it correct on my paperwork?"; "What is your date of birth?"; "What is the date today?"; "Do you have a calendar so that we can find out the date together? I must have forgotten mine."; "What do you think of the food they serve here?; "What did you have for lunch?"
  - Asking the patient to remind you when the clock reaches a certain time, as you have to check on something, make a phone call, or get to your next patient, and see if they can tell the time on their clock or watch and recall the need to remind you.
  - Asking the patient to tell you some of their medications or what time they take them, as their medication list is missing from your paperwork.
- Informal Language Assessment Examples:
  - After telling a story about yourself, asking the patient to tell you a story about themselves.
  - Asking the patient to remove certain items from your assessment bag ("Can you look in my bag and get my clipboard, please?")
  - Asking the patient how they typically spend their day or what their opinion is of the facility they are living in.
  - Asking the patient to follow 1, 2, and 3-step verbal directions about manipulating materials in the room ("Why don't we clear off this table

so that we can talk. Could you put the tissues, mail, and newspaper on the chair, please?")

- ○ Asking the patient to name items in the room or to locate and point to items you name for them.

- ○ To assess written language, having the patient assist you in making a list of items they need at the grocery store or listing tasks they may like to accomplish during the day/week.

- ○ To assess reading skills, providing the patient with the facility activity calendar, daily menu, and so forth. and asking them to read it to you. "I wonder what they're having for dinner tonight. Can you tell me?" or ask them to read part of an article in the newspaper, a piece of mail, or one of their medication bottles to assess their functional reading skills.

Informal assessment is the therapist's chance to get a little creative, so feel free to do so! Using the material within the patient's environment helps the patient to feel less anxious about "being tested" and allows you to see how the patient functions within their living space. Again, this is a great opportunity to assess the cueing needs of the patient. Can they recall the information you presented with verbal cueing? How do they respond to printed material? What are the compensatory strategies they are currently using to deal with their memory deficits? All of this information is helpful in developing a strong and individualized treatment plan.

Summary

- • Evaluation of a patient with dementia is a multifaceted process, which includes the consideration of many factors.

- • Referrals for a speech therapy evaluation for dementia may require education by the SLP to the patient's physician, payor sources, and caregivers in order to be obtained.

- • Screening is a non-billable service that can be performed for a quick assessment of a patient's deficits. Screening results may be used as justification for a referral for a full speech therapy evaluation.

- • Many areas must be considered for the evaluation of the patient with dementia, including the patient's sensory status, current health status, cultural beliefs, caregiver needs, and testing environment.

- • A thorough chart review and case history, including a patient and caregiver interview, should be included in the evaluation of a patient with dementia.

- • The evaluation process includes the use of both formal, standardized measure and informal, functional testing to obtain an accurate depiction of the patient's abilities and deficits.

References

American Speech-Language-Hearing Association (ASHA). (2005a). *The roles of speech-language pathologists working with individuals with dementia-based communication disorders: Position statement* [Position statement]. Retrieved June 30, 2013, from http://www.asha.org/policy

American Speech-Language-Hearing Association (ASHA). (2005b). *The roles of speech-language pathologists working with individuals with dementia-based communication disorders: Technical report* [Technical report]. Retrieved June 30, 2013, from http://www.asha.org/policy

Bayles, K., & Tomoeda, C. (1993). *Arizona Battery for Communication Disorders of Dementia (ABCD).* Austin, TX: Pro-Ed.

Brush, J. A., & Camp, C. J. (1998). *A therapy technique for improving memory: Spaced retrieval.* Beachwood, OH: Menorah Park Center for the Aging.

Folstein, M. F., Folstein, S. E., & McHugh, P. R. (1975). Mini-mental state: A practical method for grading the cognitive state of patients for the clinician. *Journal of Psychiatric Research, 12*(3), 189–198.

Hull, R. (1995). *Hearing in aging.* San Diego, CA: Singular.

Logsdon, R. G., Gibbons, L. E., McCurry, S. M., & Teri, L. (1999). Quality of life in Alzheimer's disease: Patient and caregiver reports. *Journal of Mental Health and Aging, 5*(1), 21–32.

Mahendra, N., & Apple, A. (2007). Assessment tools for dementia. *ASHA Leader.* Rockville, MD: American Speech-Language-Hearing Association. Retrieved from http://www.asha.org/uploadedFiles/Publications/leader/2007/071127/f071127a3.pdf

Mayo Clinic. (2011). *What is sundowning and how is it treated?* Glenn Smith (Expert opinion). Retrieved from http://www.mayoclinic.com/health/sundowning/HQ01463

Nasreddine, Z. S., Phillips, N. A., Bédirian, V., Charbonneau., S., Whitehead, V., Collin, I., . . . Chertkow, H. (2005). The Montreal Cognitive Assessment (MoCA): A brief screening tool for mild cognitive impairment. *Journal of the American Geriatrics Society, 53,* 695–699.

Randolph, C. (1998). *Repeatable Battery for the Assessment of Neuropsychological Status.* San Antonio, TX: Pearson.

Ross-Swain, D., & Fogel, P. (2011). *Ross Information Processing Assessment-Geriatric* (2nd ed.). Austin, TX: Pro-Ed.

Tariq, S., & Morley, J. (2006). *Saint Louis Mental Status Examination (SLUMS).* St. Louis, MO: Department of Veteran Affairs (VAMC).

Voeks, S., Gallagher, C., Langer, E., & Drinka, P. (1990). Hearing loss in the nursing home: An institutional issue. *Journal of the American Geriatrics Society, 38,* 141–145.

8

Goal Setting and Writing 101

You have completed your evaluation of your patient. You have several areas of deficit to work on in treatment, but where do you begin? How do you write the goals to be measure-able and achievable, as well as reimbursable by insurance providers or Medicare? You want to address not only goal areas that you believe are important to the patient's safety, functioning, and quality of life but also that have meaning to the patient, their families, and/or the staff who work with them on a daily basis, but how do you do this? This chapter focuses on developing and writing goals for patient's living with dementia. We break down the goal writing process by discussing how to prioritize goals in your treat-ment plans, incorporate patient/family/staff goals and ideas, and write goals that are explicit, easy to measure, and will get reimbursed.

Goal Writing Step One: Prioritize!

A pile of paperwork sits in front of you. Your assessments are scored; you have discussed the patient's priorities, as well as those of the family and/or the facility staff. Now what? Step one in developing a good Plan of Care for your dementia patient is to prioritize the goal areas. Before you even begin to write the goals for the patient's Plan of Care, ask yourself these questions:

1. What treatment areas will affect this person the most?
2. What means the most to the patient to address?
3. What are some abilities/strengths the patient exhibits that can help them to successfully reach their goals?

4. How many therapy sessions will you need to achieve these goals and/or how many sessions has the patient's insurance provider authorized you to have to treat this patient?

Answering these questions first will help you to see on paper how treatment of the patient should proceed. Some good rules of thumb to keep in mind as you begin the goal development process are:

1. Is the patient safe?
    *   Safety is the number one issue we should be concerned with for any patient. Safety can translate to questions such as, "Is the patient taking their medications safely and correctly?; "Is the patient able to get help if they need it?"; "Is the patient properly and consistently using equipment, such as their walker or cane?"; and "Is the patient swallowing safely?" If the patient is safe in the environment in which they live and are not at risk for harm, then you can move onto other areas of focus to address in treatment, such as communication, but safety always should be the number one priority.

2. Does the patient agree that they need therapy?
    *   This can be tricky. Sometimes the patient's family, physician, or facility staff believe the patient would benefit from speech therapy services, but the patient does not. They may not believe they have a memory problem, they may believe their issues are only a result of normal aging, or they may be nervous that by you working with them, they are admitting something is wrong and that may jeopardize their freedom and independence. As we discussed in Chapter 7, it is important during the evaluation process to explain the functions/scope of practice of the SLP and discuss that your role is to help them maintain their independence by teaching them some new or different ways to remember easier, and so forth. You need to return to how the patient feels about therapy when you are establishing goals in order to best prioritize what you will be working on with your patient. If the patient is hesitant about therapy, you will need to begin with goals that the patient mentioned as being areas they may like to work on (i.e., "I can't remember my children's names very well.") and goals that build on the patient's strengths and abilities so that they can experience success early on in treatment, see that they are capable, and look to you as someone who cares about them and is here to help them.

3. What goals will help build patient success?
    *   It is important to start with goals that are not the most difficult for the patient to achieve. As stated above, you want the patient to experience success early on in treatment to build their self-confidence and to help build and establish a rapport with you as their therapist. Starting treatment with a goal or goals that will be difficult for the patient to address may result in that patient becoming frustrated and not wanting to participate in therapy.

Ease into the treatment process. Starting with meaningful goals that are likely to be achieved will pave the way for successfully working on more difficult goals in the future.

Anatomy of a Goal

If you have been a practicing SLP for a while, you are all too familiar with writing goals. If you are a new therapist, this can be an area that can be quite tricky and can lead to quite a bit of stress until you become more comfortable with the process. In general, however, it is important for all of us, new and more seasoned SLPs alike, to review the process of writing a strong goal. Now more than ever, it is imperative to make sure our goals are written to be both measureable and attainable, along with being explicit as to what you are addressing and why, in order to get reimbursed for payment by insurance or Medicare. A goal also must be functional, meaning that addressing it will affect the patient's overall level of functioning and quality of life. So let us walk through the key elements of a goal:

A strong goal needs to be:

1. Measureable

   - Every goal needs to include how you will measure attainment. This can include percentage of trials or time (e.g., 90% of trials; 80% of meals) or be more specific to number of trials or time (e.g., eight out of ten trials, three times during 5-minute period). Determining how you will measure the goal is specific to the type of goal you are addressing. For example, a goal for a patient working on using a chin tuck position during meals to reduce aspiration risk may use the percentage of trials the chin tuck is used by the patient during meals to measure attainment.

   "Patient will recall and demonstrate use of the chin tuck position when swallowing during meals 80% trials with minimal verbal cueing to reduce risk of aspiration."

   Using the percentage of trials to measure this goal makes sense because the number of swallows during a given meal will vary, so measuring by use of the chin tuck by percentage will be much easier to document over time. In order to determine how high to set the level of attainment, you will need to return to the patient's assessment and evaluation results to see where the patient functioned at baseline with the skill and set a level that is likely to be attainable and functional for the patient. We address this further below.

2. Attainable

   - As just stated, it is important for each goal you write and set to be attainable and achievable by the patient and/or family. Again, you will want to revisit the patient's assessment results to determine what will signify attainment of each goal. You also will need to determine if the goal is realistic to achieve in the time you have to treat the patient and taking into account other factors, such as the patient's and family's motivation for treatment, likely follow through and practice outside of therapy sessions, and the patient's overall health status, as all of these will impact the likelihood of the goal being achieved or not.

3. Explicit
   - Many times the people reading the goals set by the SLP are not speech pathologists themselves. They may be physicians, families, other disciplines, or insurance companies. These people are not likely to have a working knowledge of our discipline or the terminology we use, as well as perhaps not understanding how or why we are addressing a goal in the first place. This is very apparent when working with patients with dementia, as many still mistakenly believe that these patients cannot learn or recall any new information and therefore are not likely to benefit from skilled therapy services. When writing goals for dementia patients, then, we must be explicit in why we are addressing each goal so that someone who is unfamiliar with the patient and speech therapy in general will understand what we are doing and why we are doing it. We address this further in "Chapter 11: Documentation: Connecting the Dots" related to daily treatment notes and progress reports, but it is important to mention here as we discuss the elements needed for a strong, reimbursable goal.

4. Functional
   - One of the most important elements of any well-written goal, especially ones written for dementia clients, is that the goal be functional. This means that goal should make sense to address in therapy to help the patient perform something meaningful to them in their daily life. This can include areas such as recalling their room number in the facility they live in so that they can locate their room without assistance, knowing how to locate and use emergency numbers within their home if they need help, or properly using a list of medications to identify their pills and adhere to their medication schedule in order to remain independent at home. Functional goals also can be written for staff and family members. Examples may include having the family be able to teach-back to you aspiration prevention measures or staff demonstrating how to properly thicken a patient's liquids to a recommended consistency.

Additional Elements of a Strong Goal

Include Conditions

Along with a goal being measureable, attainable, and explicit, a well-written goal also should include the conditions under which the goal will be attained. This includes the amount and level of cueing provided (e.g., minimal cueing, moderate cueing, maximal cueing or independently) and by whom (e.g., you (the therapist), facility staff member, family member, by the patient themselves) and the type of cueing provided (e.g., visual, verbal, tactile, auditory).

Use of Understandable Language

As previously stated, it is important for us to use terminology in our goals that is understandable to someone who in not familiar with our field. We want to paint a picture of who the patient is and why we are addressing each goal within the goal. This means staying away from overuse of professional terminology or explaining such terminology within the goal. For example, if we were writing a goal focused on use of compensatory strategies for a patient to improve naming and identifying items in their environment, we would want to state what these compensatory strategies are within the goal.

"Patient will utilize compensatory strategies, such as describing an item by function and/or attributes or stating the initial letter of an item, eight out of ten trials with minimal verbal cueing to improve expression of wants and needs."

This goal defines what a compensatory strategy is and what specific strategies we will be using to help the patient better express himself/herself.

Beyond being aware of using less difficult words to explain professional language in goal writing, it also is important to utilize verbiage in the goal that is measureable. This means staying away from words like "understand," "know," and "comprehend," as these are difficult to measure to determine goal attainment. Words such as "answer," "demonstrate," and "explain" are much more explicit and easier to measure.

Short-Term and Long-Term Goals

It is important to briefly discuss the difference between a short-term and long-term goal here, as both will need to be included in the dementia patient's plan of care. Long-term goals cover an extended period of treatment intervention (e.g., a Medicare certification period, in-patient rehabilitation stay) and state what you ultimately would like to see the patient achieve during that time. Short-term goals state the steps the patient will take to achieve the long-term goal and allow measurement of the patient's response to intervention and prognosis for meeting the long-term goal. Our focus thus far has been on the development of short-term goals, but all rules stated also apply to the development and writing of long-term goals. Here is an example of both short-term and long-term goals for a home health care patient in speech therapy.

Long-Term and Short-Term Goals Case Study

The patient is a home healthcare client who has dementia and recently was provided with a walker for safe ambulation. Physical therapy reports that the patient often forgets that he has the walker and often is found walking around the house without it, increasing his fall risk and risk for injury. A speech therapy order was obtained to address memory and safety in using the walker.

Long-Term Goals

1. By the end of the Medicare certification period, patient will recall and demonstrate safe use of walker to ambulate independently in home and reduce fall risk.

Short-Term Goals

1. Patient will recall need for walker to safely ambulate at the initial trial of three consecutive therapy sessions using the Spaced Retrieval technique (technique to improve memory/recall in persons with cognitive impairments).

2. Patient will recall and regularly utilize walker correctly when ambulating in home eight out of ten trials independently.

Goal Examples

For many of our patients with dementia, the top areas of treatment fall into three categories: Communication, Oral Intake, and Cognition. Here we will provide examples of goals from each of these categories to serve as a jumping-off point for developing more individualized and specific goals for your patients. It is not recommended that you use these goals verbatim when developing your treatment plans but to use them as inspiration when determining what goals make the most sense for you to use with each individual patient. You may need to alter the cueing level stated, the achievement/attainment level, or the reasoning as to why you are addressing each goal based on each case. However, we all need a little help from time to time and it is our hope that the goals shared here can provide you with some initial ideas of where to begin when working with specific treatment areas with your patients with dementia.

Communication Goals

As speech pathologists, one of our most important areas of concern when treating patients in any setting is improving their ability to communicate with others and/or help the people who care for them communicate more easily with our patients. It is important to note again that many of our patients with dementia not only are living with the symptoms of dementia but also may be living with the effects of other diseases as well, such as Parkinson's disease, stroke, dysarthria, respiratory issues, and so forth. The goals listed below are some examples of goals that focus on treating communication in persons with dementia but that also may address additional treatment areas related to communication deficits seen with other diseases that coexist with dementia.

1. Patient will demonstrate increased word recall skills to improve overall expression of wants and needs by utilizing compensatory strategies, such as

description and/or use of synonyms, 80% of trials with minimal verbal and visual cueing.

2. Patient will locate and use target communication word cards, stating common wants/needs, to improve communication with facility staff eight out of ten trials with minimal verbal cueing.

3. Patient will correctly utilize pain assessment chart, depicting areas of the body that are in pain and level of pain severity, nine out of ten trials with minimal verbal cueing to assist caregivers in addressing pain management needs.

4. Patient will correctly locate and read labeled items in room to improve word recall skills and increase participation in self-care nine out of ten trials with minimal verbal cueing.

5. Client will recall and demonstrate use of strategy of taking deeper breaths prior to speaking to promote increased volume and subglottal pressure and increase understanding by listeners 90% of trials with moderate verbal cues.

6. Client will recall and demonstrate proper placement of articulators (i.e., tongue, lips, teeth) to produce alveolar sounds (e.g., /t/, /d/, /n/, /s/, and /z/) at word level to increase communication abilities and intelligibility of speech 80% of trials with minimal verbal and visual cueing.

7. Patient will demonstrate the ability to choose between two items on a written list to communicate wants/needs related to meal, self-care, and leisure eight out of ten trials with minimal verbal cueing.

8. Patient will correctly utilize established alternative communication device to express daily wants/needs 90% of trials with moderate verbal cueing and physical demonstration.

9. Patient will read and follow written script to participate in telephone conversations to improve interaction with family and friends eight out of ten trials with minimal verbal cueing.

10. Patient will utilize picture board to identify needs related to activities of daily living (ADLs) and social interaction eight out of ten trials with moderate verbal cueing and physical demonstration.

Oral Intake Goals

Oral intake and swallowing issues become more and more prevalent with the aging population and often are one of the top areas of referral for SLPs working with older adults. Below are some examples of goals addressing directly with patients safe oral intake of foods and liquids, use of compensatory swallow strategies to decrease risk of choking and/or aspiration, and working with caregivers of dementia patients on these areas as well. You will note that many of the goals include use of a visual cue, such as a note card with written reminders to be placed in front of the client during eating, to increase the patient's recall of swallowing recommendations while eating.

1. Patient will recall and demonstrate use of chin tuck strategy when swallowing during meals 80% of trials to decrease risk of aspiration with use of visual cue and minimal verbal cueing.

2. Patient will demonstrate use of reduced bite size 80% of trials during meals using adaptive equipment and minimal verbal cueing to reduce risk of choking.

3. Patient will demonstrate decreased rate of eating during meals by placing utensil on plate between bites 90% of trials during meals using visual cue and minimal verbal cueing to reduce choking risk.

4. Patient will recall and demonstrate use of double swallows following each bite of food 80% of trials during 5-minute intervals during meals to reduce risk of aspiration.

5. Patient will demonstrate decreased pocketing of food in oral cavity by recalling to sweep oral cavity with tongue following each bite of food 80% of trials during meals using a visual cue and moderate verbal cueing and physical demonstration.

6. Patient will recall and demonstrate use of liquid wash following every two bites of food to increase hydration and decrease choking risk 80% of trials with use of visual cue and minimal verbal cueing.

7. Caregivers will demonstrate ability to teach-back elements of established aspiration prevention program with 90% accuracy.

8. Caregivers will recall and demonstrate proper thickening of liquids to honey consistency two out of three trials during three consecutive sessions to decrease patient's risk of aspiration.

9. Caregivers will demonstrate proper cleaning of patient's oral cavity to reduce colonization of bacteria in mouth and reduce aspiration risk during three consecutive therapy sessions.

10. Caregivers will demonstrate proper meal setup of patient's food, including types of food prepared, cutting to safe bite size, and positioning on plate to increase patient's amount of oral intake and ability to self-feed during three consecutive therapy sessions.

Cognition Goals

With many clients with dementia, working on cognitive goals, including memory, is a key area of focus in skilled speech therapy treatment. Many of the goals listed below rely on use of visual cueing and repeated practice of the goal areas in order for carryover to occur. A goal still can be considered to be attained if the patient can recall the information through use of a visual or written reminder. Using written reminders often is the best way to insure that the goal will be maintained following discharge from service, as the patient's memory skills will continue to decline over time due to the progressive nature of dementia. You also will note the use of the Spaced Retrieval technique in these goals, which is a technique that has been shown to help persons with cognitive impairment recall information over progressively longer intervals of time (Bourgeois et al., 2003). Discussion of Spaced Retrieval technique is given in Chapter 9. We also have listed below some goals that are focused on addressing behavioral challenges that often are seen with the dementia population. These challenges often are a source of great caregiver stress and can be addressed with a skilled service, such as speech therapy, as long as documentation of the regular occurrence of the behaviors is made either by facility staff, such as in nursing notes, or in your initial evaluation of the patient as an area of need for the patient and caregivers. We discuss this further in "Chapter 11: Documentation: Connecting the Dots" and "Chapter 12: Behavioral Issues."

1. Patient will recall times of medication administration using visual cue to increase medication adherence during three consecutive therapy sessions using the Spaced Retrieval technique (technique used to help persons recall information over progressively longer intervals of time).

2. Patient will demonstrate proper self-administration of medications by taking medications at correct dosage times as evidenced by use of medication checklist and assessment of patient's medication organizer to insure medication adherence during three consecutive therapy sessions.

3. Patient will correctly recall facility room number to decrease wandering in facility and increase overall safety during three consecutive therapy sessions using the Spaced Retrieval technique (technique used to help persons recall information over progressively longer intervals of time).

4. Patient will recall and demonstrate ability to read facility staff name badges in order to identify caregivers eight out of ten trials with minimal verbal cueing.

5. Patient will recall need to ambulate with walker at all times to decrease fall risk using visual cues at the initial trial of three consecutive therapy sessions using the Spaced Retrieval technique (technique used to help persons recall information over progressively longer intervals of time).

6. Patient will recall and demonstrate recommended hip precautions to reduce risk of re-injury using a visual cue eight out of ten trials.

7. Patient will recall location of personal memory book and use book in order to better remember personal information and daily routines during three consecutive sessions using the Spaced Retrieval technique (technique used to help persons recall information over progressively longer intervals of time).

8. Patient will recall location of emergency numbers in home and read list aloud in order to increase safety within home eight out of ten trials with minimal verbal cueing.

9. Patient will recall and utilize medication administration checklist in order to recall taking medications and decrease repetitive question asking behavior

to facility staff during three consecutive therapy sessions using the Spaced Retrieval technique (technique used to help persons recall information over progressively longer intervals of time).

10.   Patient will utilize visual cue in order to recall telephone conversations with family to decrease agitation and frequency of calls to family 80% of trials.

Case Study

Let us now attempt to put this all together! Below is a case study of a patient with dementia living in a long-term care facility, listing patient background, assessment findings, and caregiver feedback. Following this information, Figure 8–1 documents the process of establishing this patient's speech therapy goals. The guidelines provided to develop the goals also may be found in the Appendix of this book under "Goal Development Worksheet." We recommend using this worksheet with each patient you see to develop efficient, functional, and effective treatment plans.

R. T. is an 82-year-old male living in a long-term care facility. Diagnoses include dementia, congestive heart failure, asthma, and type 2 diabetes. R. T. is a former autoworker whose wife is deceased. He has four children who all live out of town. His therapy will be covered under his Medicare Part B benefit. His assessment results include a score of 13 out of 30 on the Mini-Mental Status Evaluation (MMSE; Folstein, Folstein, & McHugh, 1975); able to read 48 pt. sized Arial font; client passed Spaced Retrieval Screen (Bourgeois et al., 2003). Patient stated in evaluation that he was open to receiving therapy, although he stated that he "didn't think it would do much good."

- Client Input: Client wants to do more "on his own" and does not enjoy being around "all of the sick people." Feels "bored" and misses his family and old way of life.

- Staff Input: Resident often is found napping in other residents' rooms; often leaves cane in room; tends to take large bites of food when eating, leading to choking; wears cologne, sometimes in "excessive amounts"

- Family Input: Satisfied with care; would like a way to communicate with their father and update him on family events beyond talking on the phone.

Figure 8–1 helps to develop a systematic "plan of attack" when working with this patient. By completing the steps listed on the "Goal Development Worksheet," a therapist easily can see what the priority levels for treatment are and then can plot out the patient's treatment in a meaningful way. Additional goals also can be added if the original goals are met or need to be changed during the course of treatment. For this patient, this may include developing a way for the patient's children to communicate with him more effectively or activity recommendations that can be made to help keep the patient engaged, "less bored," and happier in the facility environment.

Goal Development Worksheet

Patient Name/Initials: R.T.

Diagnoses: Dementia, CHF, asthma, type 2 diabetes

Payor/Insurance: Medicare Part B

# of Sessions Authorized/Anticipated Length of Treatment: 3 times a week for 4 weeks

Does Patient Agree With Need for Treatment? _√_Y __N

Summary of Assessment Results: 13/30 MMSE; reads 48 pt. size Arial font; passed spaced retrieval screen

Patient/Caregiver Feedback:
Pt. wants to do more "on his own" and doesn't enjoy being around "all of the sick people". Feels "bored" and misses his family

Staff: Pt. naps in other rooms; leaves cane in room; takes large bites of food (choking); wears lots of cologne.

Family: Satisfied with care; communicate with beyond talking on phone

Does Patient Agree With Need for Treatment? _√_Y __N

Patient Strengths/Abilities:
1. Likes to "help out"
2. Functional reading/writing skills
3. Friendly but shy

Patient Personal Goals:
1. Be less bored; feel needed

2. Not fall again

3. Recall personal info better

Family/Caregiver Goals:
1. **Staff:** Decrease behavior issues/increase safety

2. **Family:** Feel closer to their dad

Is Patient Safe in Environment?
__Y _√_N
Fall risk (not using cane); choking risk

Can Patient Communicate Wants/Needs? _√_Y __N

Is Patient Eating Safely? __Y _√_N
Choking risk; large bites of food

Priority Areas of Treatment:
1. Use of cane
2. Reduced bite size of food
3. Orientation (room location)

Goals That Will Likely Lead to Early Success
1. Use of cane (fear of falling)

2. Finding room

3. Use of memory book to recall personal info

Figure 8–1. Goal development worksheet. *continues*

Goal Development Worksheet, continued

Long-Term Goal/s: *By the* *end of 12 treatment sessions,* **the patient will**

1. Recall and demonstrate safe use of cane to ambulate independently in facility and reduce fall risk.

2. Recall and demonstrate safe bite size while eating to reduce choking risk.

3. Recall facility room number to reduce wandering behaviors.

4. Use memory book to locate and recall personal information/routines.

Short-Term Goal/s: *Patient will:*
Do What?   How Often?   Why?   Conditions?

1. Recall reasons for needing cane at the beginning of 3 consecutive tx sessions using Spaced Retrieval technique to increase use of cane & reduce fall risk with use of visual cues.

2. Recall and demonstrate regular use of cane outside of room 80% of trials during treatment sessions and via staff report to reduce fall risk with minimal verbal cues.

3. Demonstrate use of smaller bite size while eating 80% of trials during meals with use of visual cue and minimal verbal cueing.

4. Correctly recall facility room number and locate room independently to reduce wandering during 3 consecutive tx sessions using the Spaced Retrieval technique.

5. Read and utilize personal memory book to recall important personal information and daily routines 80% of trials with minimal verbal cueing.

Caregiver Goal/s: *Caregiver(s) will:*
Do What?   How Often?   Why?   Conditions?

1. Provide verbal cueing to patient as instructed by SLP to assist patient in recalling need and use of cane to reduce fall risk as evidenced by patient regularly using cane.

2. Place visual cue in front of patient at all meals to increase adherence to swallowing safety program to reduce pt. choking risk at all meals during 1 week period.

3. Verbally cue patient to recall facility room number and memory book per SLP instructions as evidenced by patient recalling both when asked at random.

Figure 8–1. *continued*

Summary

- Before attempting to set goals for a patient with dementia, it is important to prioritize the goals. It is important to look at patient safety, goals that are directly meaningful to the patient, what abilities and strengths the patient has that you can utilize in your treatment to impact success, and how many sessions you need to complete treatment. This may be dictated by the number of visits authorized by the patient's insurance.

- It also is important to answer the questions, "Is the patient safe?"; "Does the patient believe they need therapy?"; and "What goals will help build patient success?" when establishing a treatment plan for your patients.

- All goals should be measureable, attainable, explicit, and functional, and include conditions and understandable language.

- Long-term and short-term goals are critical pieces of a patient's treatment plan.

- Goals for dementia patients typically fall into one of three categories: communication, oral intake, and cognition.

- A well thought-out treatment plan can lead to a structured plan of attack when working with your patients. Taking the time to establish well-written and meaningful goals will benefit not only the patient but also you and the patient's caregivers in the long run.

References

Bourgeois, M., Camp, C., Rose, M., White, B., Malone, M., Carr, J., & Rovine, M. (2003). A comparison of training strategies to enhance use of external aids by persons with dementia. *Journal of Communication Disorders, 36*(5), 361–378.

Folstein, M. F., Folstein, S. E., & McHugh, P. R. (1975). Mini-mental state: A practical method for grading the cognitive state of patients for the clinician. *Journal of Psychiatric Research, 12*(3), 189–198.

CHAPTER

9

Treatment Trends

The assessments are scored. The goals are written. Now we must decide how to proceed with treatment for a patient with dementia. There are many suggested approaches to structuring treatment, ranging from direct approaches with the patient to address memory, problem solving, and communication, to programs/recommendations to use with the patient's caregivers. This chapter summarizes the current treatment trends with patients with dementia and examples of these approaches to help in choosing the ones that best will fit your patient's needs and the needs of the people who help to care for them.

The Spaced Retrieval Technique

The Spaced Retrieval (SR) technique has been referred to earlier in this manual regarding screening and goal development. Here we will discuss the specifics of the technique and how it can be used to help a patient with dementia reach their therapeutic goals.

First noted by Landauer and Bjork in 1978, SR refers to a technique that allows for the practice of recalling information over progressively longer intervals of time. SR has been studied with numerous populations, including persons with cerebrovascular accident (CVA) (Fridriksson, Holland, Beeson, & Morrow, 2005), persons with traumatic brain injury (TBI) (Turkstra & Bourgeois, 2005), persons with human immunodeficiency virus (HIV) (Lee & Camp, 2001; Neundorfer et al., 2004), persons with Parkinson's disease (Hayden & Camp, 1995), and persons with dementia (Bourgeois et al., 2003; Brush & Camp, 1998). We suggest that the reader review the many research articles available related to the SR technique for a full explanation of the technique and its validity in use with different populations. For the purposes of this manual, the basic structure of the SR technique is to ask a patient a prompt question related to the goal area you are addressing and teach the patient a response to the prompt question (Brush & Camp, 1998; Hopper et al., 2005). The technique then requires an immediate recall of the target response from the patient,

83

and then time intervals between practices of the patient recalling the response to the prompt question are systematically lengthened until the patient can recall the response/target behavior in everyday situations. For example, let us say you are seeing a patient who is having trouble recalling the name of his daughter. The prompt question for SR training may be, "What is your daughter's name?" The target response to this question may be, "Mary." The clinician would instruct the patient on the SR technique and the target response as follows.

> *"Today we are going to work together to help you remember your daughter's name more easily. When I ask you, 'What is your daughter's name?,' I'd like you to say, 'Mary.' Let's try this."*
>
> *Clinician: "What is your daughter's name?"*
>
> *Patient response: "Mary."*
>
> *"Good! We are going to practice this for a while today. Each time I ask you, 'What is your daughter's name?,' I'd like you to say, 'Mary.'"*

Here the clinician is instructing the patient on what the prompt question and target response are, as well as asking the patient to demonstrate immediate recall of the information when asked the prompt question. Once immediate recall of the information is established, the clinician extends the time interval between asking the prompt question so that the patient can demonstrate recall of the information over extended intervals of time. For example, related to the scenario above, the clinician would proceed with SR training by doing the following:

Approximately 10 seconds after the immediate recall trial, the clinician then would ask the same prompt question again to the patient. Ten seconds after prompt question asked, Clinician: "What is your daughter's name?" Patient: "Mary." Clinician: "Great! We're going to continue practicing today." The clinician then would systematically extend the time interval before asking the prompt question again. In this case, the clinician then would ask the prompt question again 30 seconds later. If the patient successfully recalls the target response of "Mary" at the 30-second time interval, the clinician then would wait approximately one minute (twice as long as 30 seconds), then ask the prompt question again. With each correct response from the patient, the time intervals between recall trials become longer. After demonstrating recall at one minute, the clinician then would extend the time interval to 2 minutes, then 4 minutes, then 8 minutes, and so forth, thus extending the amount of time the patient is recalling the target information.

If at any time the patient cannot successfully recall the target information, the clinician provides the patient with the correct response, asks the prompt question again, has the patient respond with the target response, and then returns to the time interval at which the patient last demonstrated successful recall. For example:

> *At the two-minute time interval, the patient is asked, "What is your daughter's name?" and the patient responds, "I can't remember." The clinician then would say, "Your daughter's name is Mary. What is your daughter's name?" If the patient*

responds with the correct response of "Mary," the clinician then would wait approximately one minute and ask the prompt question again, thus returning to the last time interval where the patient demonstrated successful recall (one minute). Spaced Retrieval training then would continue from the one-minute time interval, extending or reducing the time between the asking of the prompt question based on the patient's demonstration of successful recall.

Bjork (1988) referred to SR as a form of shaping applied to memory, in that the ultimate goal of using the technique is recall of information over clinically meaningful periods of time (e.g., days, weeks, months). Brush and Camp (1998) explain that "the lengthening of time intervals represents closer and closer approximations of the ultimate goal of training," meaning that extending the length of time between practice of recalling the target information allows for systematic practice of recall, helping the patient get closer to recalling the information for meaningful lengths of time, such as days, weeks, and months. Use of SR can be clinically relevant then for use in treating patients with dementia, as our goal for working with these patients is to improve their recall ability for important information for meaningful periods of time with the goal of improving their overall safety and level of functioning.

As briefly discussed in Chapter 7, there is a screening approach that can be used to assess if a patient is a candidate for benefitting from SR training. The Screening Form can be found in Brush and Camp (1998) and can be described as being a sort of "mini spaced retrieval session." The SR screen assesses a patient's ability to recall a given piece of information, such as the clinician's name, during three progressively longer time intervals (immediate recall, short delay (10 to 15 seconds, and long delay (20 to 30 seconds). If the patient is able to demonstrate recall of the target information at each time interval, he/she is considered to be a good candidate for use of the technique in therapy. If the patient is unable to recall the target information at any of the time intervals in the screening measure, the patient is provided with the target response, asked the prompt question again ("What is my name?"), asked to provide the target response again, and then testing is returned to the last time interval where the patient demonstrated successful recall of the information (immediate recall or short delay). The patient has three opportunities at each time interval to demonstrate recall. If the patient is unable to recall the information at the long recall interval for three opportunities, he/she is not considered to be a good candidate for SR training. We recommend incorporating the "Spaced Retrieval Screen" into every evaluation of a patient with dementia. This will allow you, as the clinician, to know if the patient can benefit from this sort of training in therapy to help the patient reach his/her goals.

Examples of Spaced Retrieval Goal Areas, Prompts, and Responses

Because Spaced Retrieval is a technique for teaching information and improving recall of information, it has many applications to working with the dementia population.

Some examples of treatment goals and prompt questions/responses where SR may be useful are below. Additional examples of goals using SR can be found in Chapter 8 of this manual.

- **Treatment Goal:** Recall of facility room number or home address; Prompt Question: "What is your room number (address)?" Response: Correct room number or home address

- **Treatment Goal:** Recall of need for walker to ambulate safely; Prompt Question: "What do you need with you any time you walk?" Response: "My walker"

- **Treatment Goal:** Recall of use of chin tuck when swallowing to prevent aspiration risk; Prompt Question: "What should you do when you swallow?" Response: "Tuck my chin (or look at my lap)"

- **Treatment Goal:** Recall of use of description to decrease anomia; Prompt Question: "If you don't know the name of something, what should you do?" Response: "Describe it"

- **Treatment Goal:** Recall of use of medication timer and response to timer to improve medication adherence; Prompt Question: "What should you do when you hear the loud beep?" Response: "Take my pills"

- **Treatment Goal:** Recall of steps to complete daily routines/activities of daily living (ADLs); Prompt Question: "Where should you look to remember what you need to do in the morning?" Response: "The checklist on my mirror"

Additional Considerations for Spaced Retrieval

The limits of what you can teach a patient to recall using SR really are limited only to the creativity and imagination of the clinician. It should be noted that the information/strategies trained using SR should be meaningful to the patient in order to insure greater recall and retention of the information. Asking the patient what they would like to remember better during the evaluation process will help in the development of meaningful SR goals. Also, incorporating the patient's language and/or routines into the training goals/sessions is helpful, meaning that if you as the clinician would like the patient to recall using a memory book to recall personal information, you should ask the patient what they themselves would call the memory book. The patient may refer to the memory book as "my scrapbook" or "my photo album." You then would incorporate the patient's term for the memory book into the target response for the patient's SR prompt question (i.e., Prompt Question: "What should you look at to better remember your family?" Response: "My scrapbook").

Incorporating recall of information into the patient's normal routines also will assist with carryover of the SR goal, meaning if the SR goal is focused on the patient recalling to put hearing aids in his/her ears each morning, you would want to incorporate recall of this behavior into how the patient normally gets ready in the morning (i.e., Prompt Question: "What should you do after you brush your teeth?" Response: "Put in my hearing aids"). Discussion with the patient and/or the patient's caregivers regarding regular routines is recommended during the evaluation and treatment process to assist in the overall carryover of the goals.

Spaced Retrieval can be incorporated in the patient's treatment sessions to address a number of goals. During the time intervals between recall trials, the clinician can address an additional goal or goals, participate in conversation with the client, or work on a meaningful activity with the client, such as looking at family pictures, performing ADLs, and so forth (Hinckley, Bourgeois, & Hickey, 2011).

Progress on goals using the SR technique is measured by length of time the patient can successfully recall the target information and/or show regular demonstration of a target behavior, such as the patient regularly recalling to tuck his/her chin when swallowing, regularly locating his/her room with minimal to no assistance, or safely using his/her walker on a regular basis. Brush and Camp (1998) recommend that at the beginning of each subsequent therapy session after SR training begins, the clinician asks the patient the prompt question for the goal area they are addressing to see if the patient has retained the information since the last treatment session. Most of the time this constitutes a time interval of anywhere from 24 to 48 hours. If the patient can recall the information at the beginning of a subsequent treatment session, the clinician does not need to address this goal further during that session. If the patient can demonstrate successful recall of the target information/behavior during three consecutive therapy sessions, the goal can be considered attained. It is recommended, however, that the clinician make sure the patient is regularly following through with recalling the information/behavior in meaningful contexts, meaning that the patient not only is able to tell you that he needs his walker when he walks but also is actually using his walker when he walks. The best way to make sure this carryover occurs is to regularly practice use and demonstration of the target information in the patient's therapy session. This translates, for example, not only to teaching the patient his/her room number in treatment using SR but also to incorporating the patient practicing using the information to locate his/her room as part of your treatment session with him/her.

If the patient is unable to recall the target response at the beginning of a subsequent treatment session, Brush and Camp (1998) recommend that the clinician provide the patient with the correct response to the prompt question, ask the prompt question again, have the patient respond with the correct response, and then return to last time interval the patient reached in the previous treatment session. For example, if the patient was able to recall the target response for up to 8 minutes during the previous treatment session and was unable to correctly recall the response at the beginning of the subsequent treatment session, the clinician then would wait eight minutes before asking the prompt question again in the subsequent session to resume training at the highest time interval the patient was able to achieve previously.

Once a patient reaches his/her goal using SR, the SLP can instruct the patient's caregivers on use of the prompt question with the patient within the patient's everyday life. The prompt question and response also can be written into the patient's discharge plan or facility plan of care to insure follow-through and carryover of the goal.

Montessori-Based Dementia Programming®

Another treatment strategy that can be used with patients with dementia is Montessori-Based Dementia Programming® (MBDP). Developed and researched by Camp and colleagues (Camp et al., 1997; Orsulic-Jeras, Camp, Lee, & Judge, 2005; Skrajner, Malone, Camp, McGowan, & Gorzelle, 2007), MBDP uses Montessori educational principles to help persons with physical and/or cognitive impairments participate more effectively in activities in their everyday lives. MBDP has been used effectively with both individuals (Camp et al., 1997) and groups (Skrajner & Camp, 2004) and can be used by SLPs to better structure activities during treatment sessions and in educating caregivers and facility staff on how to more effectively work with their loved ones/patients with dementia. We again recommend that a thorough review of the literature related to the research of use of Montessori methods with persons with dementia be conducted by the clinician prior to using this method in treatment. There also are a number of instructional/activity manuals available describing Montessori-based activities and their application to persons with dementia that are useful additions to the speech pathologist's library (Camp, 1999; Camp et al., 2006; Joltin, Camp, Noble, & Antenucci, 2005).

Camp (1999) describes some key principles to using Montessori methods with persons with dementia. The SLP can utilize these principles in their practice to improve the patient's participation in treatment activities and in creating treatment activities that are meaningful in helping a patient reach his/her therapeutic goals. Some of these key principles include:

- Using real-life materials that are aesthetically pleasing
- Progressing from the simple to the complex
- Progressing from the concrete to the abstract
- Structuring materials and procedures so that the patient will work from left to right and from top to bottom (this mirrors the process of reading in Western cultures, which is a learned behavior that usually is logical and maintained in persons with dementia)
- Breaking down activities into component parts, and practicing one component at a time
- Using as little vocalization as possible when demonstrating activities
- Matching your speed of movement to the speed of movement of the patient
- Making sure that all activity materials are designed to focus attention on only one concept. Eliminate extraneous details from materials such as extra letters, numbers, or pictures on reading material as this can cause the patient to become distracted and focused on the details of the materials and not the activity itself.
- Beginning each activity with an invitation to participate and a choice of activities. It can be useful to tell the patient that you need their help to complete something, as this provides the patient with a meaningful role and reason to participate in the activity.

- When an activity is complete, asking the patient if he/she enjoyed the activity and if they would like to do it again at another time. This provides the patient with a chance to give feedback on his/her treatment and allows the therapist to gather helpful information in creating more meaningful treatment activities and/or activity recommendations for family and staff to implement with the patient.

Another key principle described by Camp and colleagues (Camp, 1999; Camp et al., 2006) is to accommodate for visual deficits when creating treatment activities/materials. They recommend use of large type (e.g., 48 or 100 point) and using a sans serif font, such as Arial or Helvetica, when utilizing print in treatment/activity materials. Use of high contrast, such as black print on a white background, also can assist the patient with visual deficits, as does the use of primary colors and texture in treatment/activity materials. Whenever possible, materials should be laminated using a nonglare laminating material to increase the visibility and durability of the materials and the ability to easily clean the materials between use to decrease the spread of germs and bacteria between patients/caregivers.

There are many examples of Montessori-based activities described in the literature and in the treatment manuals listed earlier in this chapter that can be used in speech therapy treatment sessions. The important thing the SLP should keep in mind is that any treatment material/activity can be considered Montessori-based, if the activity incorporates some of the key principles of the programming method. Therefore, recommending that the patient's clothing be laid out on their bed each morning from left to right in the order in which the patient usually puts their clothing on can assist the patient in participating more fully in getting ready in the morning and/or increase their level of independence or decrease their level of dependence on caregiver/staff assistance. This would be an example of using Montessori principles to improve treatment with a dementia patient. Creating communication cards for the patient with pictures of common wants/needs/requests, utilizing real-life pictures of the objects, large print, and no additional extraneous details on the cards would be another example of using Montessori principles in treatment. Slowly demonstrating the steps to use an augmentative communication device, using little verbalization, repetition of each step until mastered by the patient, and matching the patient's speed of movement would be another example of using Montessori methods in treatment. The possibilities of applications of this method, then, again are limited only to the creativity and imagination of the clinician.

Validation Therapy

Created by gerontological social worker, Naomi Feil (1967), Validation Therapy is "the process of communicating with a disoriented elderly person by validating and respecting their feelings in whatever time or place is real to them at the time, even though this may not correspond with our 'here and now' reality (Vanderslott, 1994, p. 151). This is in stark contrast to Reality Orientation (Hogstel, 1979), which is a commonly utilized technique by healthcare professionals. The goal of Validation Therapy is to understand the meaning behind an individual person's behavior and "validating" their beliefs (Dietch, Hewett, & Jones, 1989). Validation Therapy is classified into four different stages of disorientation, including malorientation, time confusion, repetitive motion, and vegetation (Feil, 1993). The proposed benefits of Validation Therapy include less regression inward, improved speech, reduced incidences of crying, pacing, and wandering, and reduced need for physical restraints and psychotropic medication (Feil, 1993). Although there are a number of research studies focused on use of Validation Therapy with persons with dementia (Fine & Rouse-Bane, 1995; Morton & Bleathman, 1991; Scanland & Emershaw, 1993), it still is unclear if this method has enough scientific evidence behind it to support the proposed benefits of the technique. However, it is widely used in facility settings and bears discussion in this manual as it is likely that the SLP will come in contact with it being used or discussed in facility settings. Some of the basic principles of Validation Therapy include: (a) picking up on utterances without disrupting them (using reformulation or repetition of utterances, (b) eye contact, (c) observation of body language and emotional expression, (d) use of touch, and (e) use of elements from music and Reminiscence Therapy. These techniques can be utilized as communication strategies with a patient with dementia when the patient is exhibiting a challenging behavior or expressing information or feelings that may not be true to reality or the patient's current situation but are very real to the patient, such as if a patient will not leave their room or the door to a facility because they believe they are waiting to get their children off of the school bus, even though their children are, in fact, grown. For more details on Validation Therapy and its implementation, please see the References at the end of this chapter.

Reminiscence Therapy

Reminiscence Therapy focuses on facilitating the patient with dementia to remember events or experiences in his/her life and assisting the patient in sharing these memories with others (Grasel, Wiltfang, & Kornhuber, 2003). Reminiscence Therapy often is incorporated into group discussions and uses materials such as photographs, music, and objects to stimulate recall and discussion. The goals of Reminiscence Therapy include promoting social interaction, conveying positive emotions, and promoting the self-awareness of the patient with dementia (Hodgson & Schweitzer, 1999). Reminiscence Therapy promotes the use of active listening, attentiveness to nonverbal communication signs, and use of language that is appropriate and easily understood by the patient(s) (Grasel et al., 2003). As with Validation Therapy, Reminiscence Therapy is widely used in facility settings but has little empirical evidence to support its use. However, it can be utilized by therapists and caregivers to help promote communication and social interaction with patients with dementia. Elements of Reminiscence Therapy can be used in skilled treatment to address goals such as improved self-expression, pragmatics, social skills, auditory comprehension, and attention span. Here is an example of using Reminiscence Therapy to address a goal of improved verbal expression with a patient:

Elizabeth was a former librarian at an elementary school. According to her children, Elizabeth loved her job and the children she worked with at the school. Because of Elizabeth's dementia, she has become withdrawn and her verbal output usually is limited to answering yes/no questions and simple phrases. She is being seen by speech therapy in the hopes of improving her overall verbal communication and interaction with others within the facility environment in which she lives.

Goal: "Patient will demonstrate increased verbal expression skills by using short sentences of four to five words in length related to conversational topics 80% of trials with minimal verbal cueing and demonstration to improve communication skills and social interaction with peers."

Treatment Activity: In individual therapy sessions, Elizabeth will be presented with reminiscence materials to promote recall of positive memories and improved verbal expression skills. Objects used to promote reminiscence may include library books (if possible, ones that were popular when she was working as a librarian; card catalog cards, stamp pad, and dated stamp); library cards, list of common rules of a library (e.g., "Be Quiet," "Place books back on shelf when finished," etc.). These items will be used to promote discussion and increase length of sentences with modeling from the clinician. These items then will be used in group settings of two to three patients once patient is demonstrating progress on goal in individual sessions. Additional activities for use both in therapy and outside of therapy may include placing card catalog cards in order by number, title, author, and so forth, placing book jackets on the corresponding books, and oral reading of books to others, including grandchildren, and so on.

Use of Visual/Graphic Cues and Memory Books

The use of visual/graphic cues has been widely documented as a successful treatment strategy with persons with dementia (Bourgeois, Burgio, Schulz, Beach, & Palmer, 1997; Bourgeois & Hickey, 2007, 2009). Because the ability to read appears to be somewhat maintained through the course of dementia (Bourgeois, 2001), using visual reminders/ aids can be a helpful and effective way of helping the patient with dementia compensate for their memory deficits. Using items such as index cards and memo boards (Bourgeois et al., 1997) and reminder cards (Bourgeois & Hickey, 2007) can be used to help reduce repetitive verbal behaviors in patients with dementia, which often is listed as a top caregiver stressor. Due to their limited short-term memory skills, patients with dementia may ask the same question over and over again of their caregivers, increasing the patient's anxiety and the caregiver's frustration. Using index cards to create a reminder card of the information the patient frequently asks can be an effective way of reducing this behavior. For example, if the patient often asks their loved one when their next doctor's appointment is, a reminder card stating when the next appointment is scheduled can be made and given to the patient to refer to the next time they want to recall this information. Below is an example of what this card could look like (Figure 9–1).

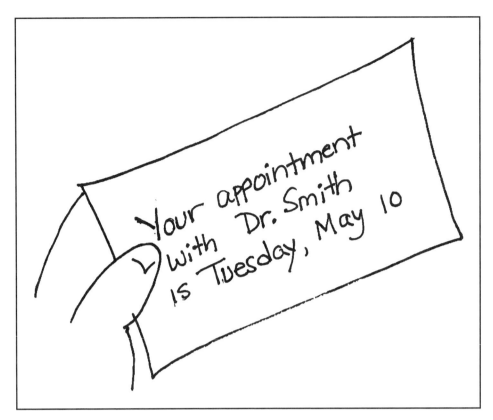

Figure 9–1. Memory card for doctor's appointment.

Reminder boards stating a patient's schedule for the day or important tasks to remember to do also can be created to compensate for the patient's decreased memory and initiation skills. A checklist of important tasks to complete or a simple statement of when a caregiver will return home from work or will be visiting the facility again can be useful reminders for the patient with decreased memory skills (Figure 9–2).

Bourgeois (2007) recommends printing a simple, clear message on visual cues, making the message personal (use of pronouns, I, you, we, etc.) and reading the message aloud prior to using it with the patient to correct for any confusion or errors.

Memory books and wallets also are useful treatment tools for the therapist working with dementia patients (Bourgeois, 1992; Bourgeois, Dijkstra, Burgio, & Allen-Burge, 2001). Memory books and wallets utilize meaningful pictures, and short, clear, concrete sentences to describe the pictures to help the patient with dementia recall important personal information, routines, and so forth. Again, the use of print to help describe a picture can help the patient with dementia compensate for the possible limited recall he/she may have for a picture or a routine and, in turn, increase their overall level of independence due to not having to rely on another person to provide this information or explanation. These tools can be kept in a person's room, walker bag, and so forth, or posted in areas where they are easily seen and accessed by the patient, such as near their bed, in their kitchen, or next to their favorite chair. Memory cards also can be attached

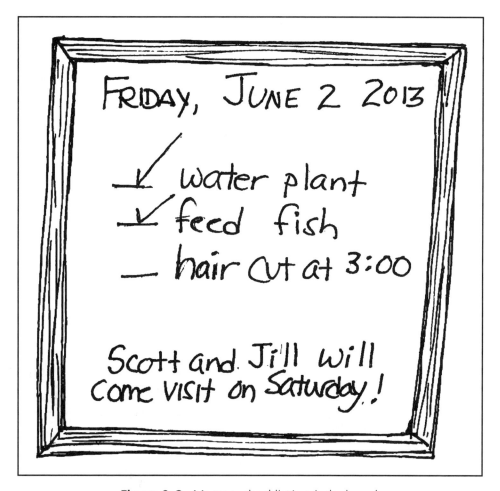

Figure 9–2. Memory checklist/reminder board.

to walkers or wheelchairs or even worn around a patient's neck or wrist to increase their accessibility and use by the patient (Bourgeois & Hickey, 2009).

Speech pathologists can use visual/graphic cues and memory books and wallets in skilled treatment to help patients reach a number of goals, such as increased communication, improved recall of personal information (e.g., room number, family member names, etc.), improved recall and adherence to routines (e.g., medication times, meal times, dietary restrictions, maintaining personal finances), and improved recall of safety information (e.g., emergency phone numbers, reminders to turn off appliances after use, such as the stove or iron, hip precautions, monitoring of blood glucose level if diabetic, use of grab bars or other adaptive equipment, and swallowing strategies). Below is an example of using visual/graphic cues in treatment with a patient with dementia.

Visual/Graphic Cues Case Study

John has early stage dementia and lives with his daughter, who works during the day. He recently has become more aware of his memory deficits, and his daughter worries about his safety when she is away from home at work. John calls his daughter frequently during the day to ask where she is and when she is returning home and about tasks that he can do around the house "to help out." John's daughter makes him lunch before she leaves for work and leaves it in the refrigerator for him to eat, but she often returns home to find the food untouched and still in the refrigerator, even though she reminds him to eat when he calls her. John's doctor recommended speech therapy via home health care to help address his memory deficits, to improve his safety, and to help his daughter better manage his care.

Speech Therapy Goals:

1. "Patient will utilize a visual cue, such as a memo board, to recall daughter's whereabouts during the day and return time home in order to improve recall and decrease multiple phone calls to daughter during day at the beginning of three consecutive therapy sessions using the spaced retrieval technique and confirmation of carryover of goal by caregiver."

2. "Patient will utilize a choice board and/or checklist to assist in choosing activities/tasks to complete during the day in order to increase engagement in activities and provide a meaningful role for patient 80% of trials."

3. "Patient will recall presence of meal in refrigerator for lunch and eat provided meal three out of five days using visual cues in order to increase nutrition and decrease risk of weight loss."

4. "Caregiver will be able to teach-back to therapist use of visual/graphic cues to assist father in recall of important personal and safety information with 90% accuracy."

Treatment Activities:

1. To address the goal of using a memo board to recall his daughter's whereabouts and return time home, the speech pathologist will create the memo board message with John and his daughter. If John is able to write and can read his own handwriting, he will be asked to write the message himself, as he will recognize his own handwriting and believe something written in his own handwriting more than if it is written in handwriting that is unfamiliar to him. If he cannot, his daughter will be asked to print the message for him with instruction from the SLP. The SR technique will be used to help John recall to read the memo board when he wants to know where his daughter is. Prompt Question: "Where do you look to find out where your daughter is and when she's coming home?" Response: "The board next to my chair." In this case, John has a favorite chair that he likes to sit in and so having the board located there will increase the chances of him using it. SR training will proceed. Once John is able to successfully recall and read the memo board at the beginning of

three consecutive sessions and the daughter reports he is using it, the goal will be considered attained (Figure 9–3).

2. To address John's willingness to complete tasks around the house and the fact that he is unsure of what to do, a choice board of activities he can do safely during the day will be made using printed words or pictures, if needed. A checklist of activities or steps to complete a given task also may be created, if needed. Treatment time will be used to create the choice board and/or checklist and to complete tasks using the visual cues with cueing and instruction from the SLP. Goal will be considered attained when John is completing 80% of the tasks on his board successfully when home alone or completing 80% of the tasks/steps listed on his checklist (Figure 9–4).

3. To address the fact that John is not aware of his lunch in the refrigerator and not eating during the day, two or more visual cues will be placed in the home in places John reports he can see them (on T.V. stand, on door frame to kitchen, bathroom mirror, and refrigerator door) reminding John that his lunch is

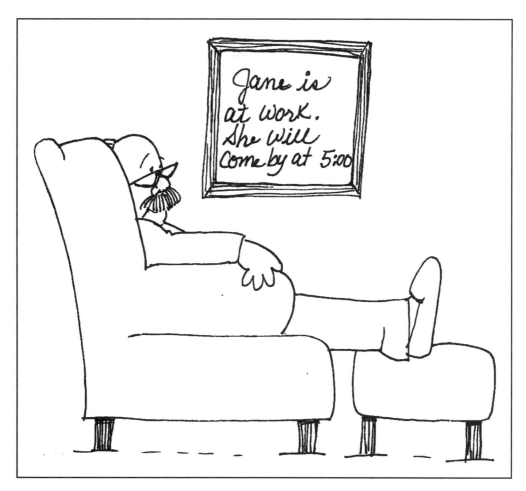

Figure 9–3. Example of memo board for case study.

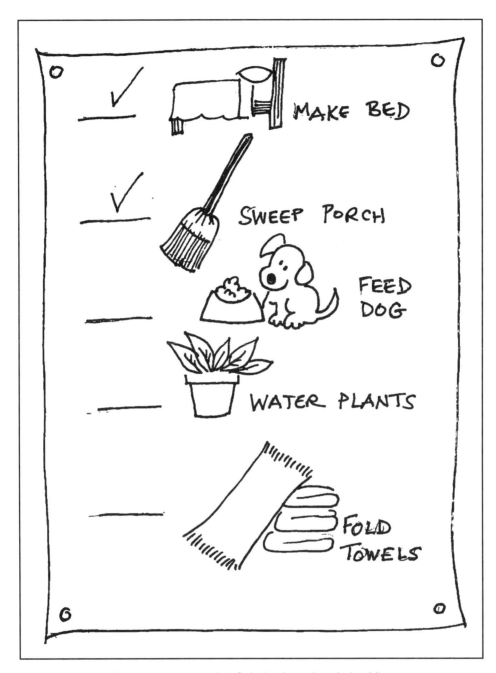

Figure 9–4. Example of choice board and checklist.

ready in the refrigerator and to eat it after the 12:00 news. Incorporating the visual cues with John's daily routine of watching the 12:00 news should help to increase his recall to get his lunch out of the refrigerator and eat it. Therapy time will be spent creating the visual cues and choosing proper and functional placement with John and his daughter (Figure 9–5). Treatment times will be scheduled around noon for at least one week in order to cue patient to read

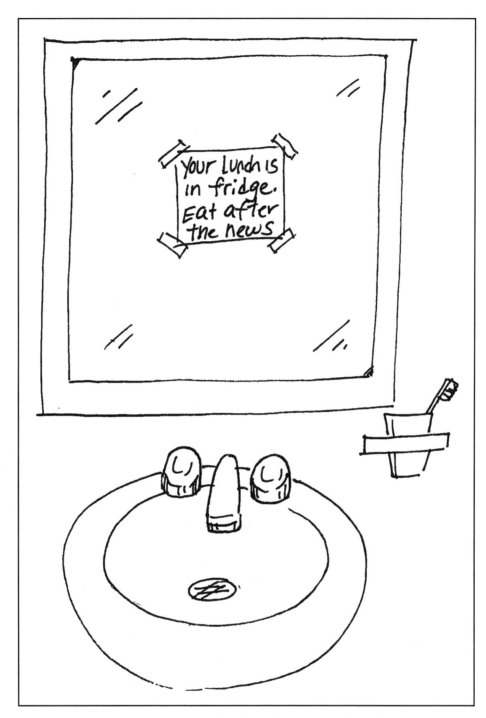

Figure 9–5. Example of visual cues to recall meal.

visual cues and to insure follow-through with strategies (i.e., eating his lunch). Goal will be considered attained when John demonstrates eating of lunch independently three out of five days as evident through caregiver report of meal being eaten and/or therapist observation.

4. To address caregiver understanding of use of visual strategies, the SLP will teach the theory behind use of visual cues with patients with dementia to compensate for memory deficits and will review key concepts such as print size, structuring of message/reminders, placement for accessibility and use of visual reminders, and cueing to recall her father to utilize them. Goal will be considered attained when the caregiver can teach-back the purpose, use, and creation of visual cues to the SLP with 90% accuracy.

Compensatory Strategies and Communication/ Conversational Approaches

The use of compensatory strategies often is cited as a critical element to treatment of the person with dementia. A compensatory strategy can be defined as an alternative means of doing something to enable success (Bourgeois & Hickey, 2009; Bayles & Tomoeda, 2007). When working with individuals with dementia, the types of compensatory strategies that can be utilized in treatment are as varied as the patients themselves. We have discussed the use of visual cues to compensate for memory/recall deficits, but additional examples can include verbal compensatory strategies, such as describing or spelling a word that cannot be recalled or asking a clarifying question to help improve understanding of information, nonverbal compensatory strategies, such as using pointing, gesturing, or facial expression to help a patient communicate wants, needs, pain, etc., when a patient is unable to do so verbally, or written compensatory strategies, such as writing down a word or using one's finger to spell a word when unable to verbally express the word. Many of these suggestions for compensatory strategies come from the research related to working with patients with aphasia (Hinckley, Bourgeois, & Hickey, 2011) but often are applicable to working with persons with dementia. In general, our goal with dementia patients is to try to circumvent the person's deficits. This means attempting to "go around the patient's memory difficulties" and use the strengths and abilities the patient has available to them to allow the patient to recall or communicate at the highest level possible. This often includes incorporating the use of some sort of compensatory strategy into the patient's treatment, as the likelihood of retaining learned information over time is reduced due to the progressive nature of dementia. Therefore, the SLP should plan on using compensatory strategies, in any form that is successful for the patient, regularly in the treatment of patients with dementia.

Strategies to increase communication and/or conversational approaches are additional treatment strategies recommended for use with patients with dementia. These strategies/approaches may include structuring conversations/interactions to utilize questions that incorporate choice (e.g., Saying, "Would you like spaghetti or pot roast for dinner tonight?" rather than, "What would you like for dinner tonight?"), or asking questions that can be answered with a simple "yes or no," and using open-ended questions that tap into the patient's semantic memory abilities (e.g., Asking, "How do you feel about the food served here?" rather than "What did you have for breakfast today?") (Hinckley,

Bourgeois, & Hickey, 2011). It has been found that the use of open-ended questions can lead to better elicitation of opinions, feelings, and even factual information (Dijkstra Bourgeois, Youmans, & Hancock, 2006; Petryk & Hopper (in press); Small & Perry, 2005; Tappen, Williams-Burgess, Edelstein, Touhy, & Fishman, 1997). Arkin (2005) describes using pros/cons to elicit conversation in persons with dementia. For example, asking the patient or group of patients the pros and cons of specific items or topics, such as visiting relatives or mandatory retirement. Dijkstra et al. (2006) suggests the use of advice or opinion scenarios to increase patient's participation in conversation. Asking questions such as, "What advice can you give me about interviewing for a job? Dealing with my in-laws? Buying a new car?" can allow the patient to express how they feel about a certain topic, while possibly triggering memories about their own personal experiences about the topic. All of these techniques for structuring conversations and asking questions not only can be incorporated into patient treatment directly by the SLP but also provided to caregivers to use during their interactions with the patients, as well.

Choosing Treatment Strategies

There is no clear-cut answer as to which treatment strategies you should use in treating patients with dementia. Many times, a good treatment plan will incorporate many of the elements of the strategies/methods discussed in this chapter. Choosing the best way to proceed with treatment with dementia patients is dependent on factors such as the types of goals you are addressing, the patient's ability to benefit from certain strategies (e.g., pass the Spaced Retrieval Screen), or the patient's additional diagnoses or physical/sensory deficits. By analyzing all of these factors and knowing the details of an intervention method, including the research evidence available to support use of the method, SLPs have many options available to proceed in creating meaningful and functional treatment plans for their patients.

Summary

- There are many treatment strategies available to the SLP working with patients with dementia, including use of the SR technique, Montessori-Based Dementia Programming®, Validation Therapy, Reminiscence Therapy, Use of Visual/Graphic Cues and Memory Books, and Compensatory and Conversational Strategies.

- Treatment not only targets working with the patient directly but also with the patient's family and/or caregivers.

- Choosing the appropriate treatment strategy for the patient with dementia is dependent on the patient's needs and goal areas. Oftentimes, elements of many of the discussed treatment strategies can be utilized in the effective treatment of these patients.

TOURO COLLEGE LIBRARY

References

Arkin, S. (2005). *Language enriched exercise for clients with Alzheimer's disease.* Tucson, AZ: Desert Southwest Fitness.

Bayles, K. A., & Tomoeda, C. K. (2007). *Cognitive-communication disorders of dementia.* San Diego, CA: Plural.

Bjork, R. A. (1988). Retrieval practice and the maintenance of knowledge. In M. M. Gruneberg, P. E. Morris, & R. N. Sykes (Eds.), *Practical aspects of memory: Current research and issues* (pp. 283–288). Chichester, UK: Wiley.

Bourgeois, M. (1992). Evaluating memory wallets in conversations with patients with dementia. *Journal of Speech and Hearing Research, 35,* 1344–1357.

Bourgeois, M. (2001). Is reading preserved in dementia? *ASHA Leader, 6*(9), 5. Rockville, MD: American Speech-Language-Hearing Association.

Bourgeois, M. (2002). Where is my wife and when am I going home? The challenge of communicating with persons with dementia. *Alzheimer's Care Quarterly, 3*(2), 132–144.

Bourgeois, M., Burgio, L., Schulz, R., Beach, S., & Palmer, B. (1997). Modifying repetitive verbalization of community dwelling patients with AD. *Gerontologist, 37,* 30–39.

Bourgeois, M., Camp, C., Rose, M., White, B., Malone, M., Carr, J., & Rovine, M. (2003). A comparison of training strategies to enhance use of external aids by persons with dementia. *Journal of Communication Disorders, 36,* 361–378.

Bourgeois, M., Dijkstra, K., Burgio, L., & Allen-Burge, R. (2001). Memory aids as an AAC strategy for nursing home residents with dementia. *Augmentative and Alternative Communication, 17,* 196–210.

Bourgeois, M., & Hickey, E. (2007). Dementia. In D. R. Beukelman, K. L. Garrett, & K. M. Yorkston (Eds.), *Augmentative communication strategies for adults with acute or chronic medical conditions* (pp. 243–285). Baltimore, MD: Brookes.

Bourgeois, M., & Hickey, E. (2009). *Dementia: From diagnosis to management—A functional approach.* New York, NY: Taylor & Francis.

Brush, J. A. & Camp, C. J. (1998). *A therapy technique for improving memory: Spaced retrieval.* Beachwood, OH: Menorah Park Center for the Aging.

Camp, C. (1999). *Montessori-based activities for persons with dementia, Volume 1.* Beachwood, OH: Menorah Park Center for Senior Living.

Camp, C., Judge, K., Bye, C., Fox, K, Bowden, J., Bell, M., . . . Mattern, J. M. (1997). An intergenerational program for persons with dementia using Montessori methods. *Gerontologist, 37,* 688–692.

Camp, C., Schneider, N., Orsulic-Jeras, S., Mattern, J., McGowan, A., Antenucci, V., . . . Gorzelle, G. (2006). *Montessori-based activities for persons with dementia: Volume 2.* Beachwood, OH: Menorah Park Center for Senior Living.

Dietch, J. T., Hewett, L. J., & Jones, S. (1989). Adverse effects of reality orientation. *Journal of the American Geriatrics Society, 37*(10), 974–976.

Dijkstra, K., Bourgeois, M., Youmans, G., & Hancock, A. (2006). Implications of an advice-giving and teacher role on language production in adults with dementia. *Gerontologist, 46*(3), 357–366.

Feil, N. (1967). Group therapy in a home for the aged. *Gerontologist, 7,* 192–195.

Feil, N. (1993). *The validation breakthrough.* Baltimore, MD: Health Professions Press.

Fine, J. I., & Rouse-Bane, S. (1995). Using validation techniques to improve communication with cognitively impaired adults. *Journal of Gerontological Nursing, 21*(6), 39–45.

Fridriksson, J., Holland, A., Beeson, P., & Morrow, L. (2005). Spaced retrieval treatment of anomia. *Aphasiology, 19*(2), 99–109.

Grasel, E., Wiltfang, J., & Kornhuber, J. (2003). Non-drug therapies for dementia: An overview of the current situation with regard to proof of effectiveness. *Dementia and Geriatric Cognitive Disorders, 15*(3), 115–125.

Hayden, C. M., & Camp, C. J. (1995). Spaced Retrieval: A memory intervention for dementia in Parkinson's disease. *Clinical Gerontologist, 16*(3), 80–82.

Hinckley, J., Bourgeois, M., & Hickey, E. (2011). *Treatments that work for both aphasia and dementia.* Presented at the annual convention of the American Speech-Language-Hearing Association, San Diego, CA.

Hodgson, B.. & Schweitzer, P. (1999). *Reminiscing with people with dementia: A handbook.* London. UK: Age Exchange.

Hogstel, M. O. (1979). Use of reality orientation with aging confused patients. *Nursing Research, 28*(3), 161–165.

Hopper, T., Mahendra, N., Kim, E., Azuma, T., Bayles, K. A., Cleary, S. J., & Tomoeda, C. K. (2005). Evidence-based practice recommendations for working with individuals with dementia: Spaced-retrieval training. *Journal of Medical Speech-Language Pathology, 13*(4), 27–34.

Joltin, A., Camp, C, Noble, B., & Antenucci, V. (2005). *A different visit: Activities for caregivers and their loved ones with memory impairments.* Beachwood, OH: Menorah Park Center for Senior Living.

Landauer, T. K., & Bjork, R. A. (1978). Optimal rehearsal patterns and name learning. In M. Grunberg, P. Morris, & R. Sykes (Eds.) *Practical aspects of memory* (pp. 625–632). London, UK: Academic Press.

Lee, M., & Camp, C. J. (2001). Spaced-retrieval: A memory intervention for HIV+ older adults. *Clinical Gerontologist, 22*, 131–135.

Morton, I., & Bleathman, C. (1991). The effectiveness of validation therapy in dementia: A pilot study. *International Journal of Geriatric Psychiatry, 6*, 327–330.

Neundorfer, M. M., Camp, C. J., Lee, M. M., Malone, M. L., Carr, J. R., & Skrajner, M. J. (2004). Compensating for cognitive deficits in persons aged 50 and over with HIV/AIDS: A pilot study of a cognitive intervention. *Journal of HIV/AIDS and Social Services, 3*(1), 79–97.

Orsulic-Jeras, S., Camp, C., Lee, M., & Judge, K. (2005). Effects of a Montessori-based intergenerational program on engagement and affect for adult day care clients with dementia. In M. L. Wykle, P. Whitehouse, & D. L. Morris (Eds.), *Successful aging through the life span: Intergenerational issues in health.* New York, NY: Springer.

Petryk, M., & Hopper, T. (in press). The effects of question type on conversational discourse in Alzheimer's disease. *Perspectives: Newsletter of the Neurophysiology and Neurogenic Special Interest Division*, American Speech-Language-Hearing Association.

Scanland, S. G., & Emershaw, L. E. (1993). Reality orientation and validation therapy: Dementia, depression, and functional status. *Journal of Gerontological Nursing, 19*(6), 7–11.

Skrajner, M., & Camp, C. (2004). Resident-Assisted Montessori Programming (RAMP): Training persons with dementia to serve as group activity leaders. *Gerontologist, 44*(3), 426–431.

Skrajner, M., Malone, M., Camp, C., McGowan, A., & Gorzelle, G. (2007). Research in practice: Montessori-based dementia programming. *Alzheimer's Care Quarterly, 8*(1), 53–64.

Small, J., & Perry, J. (2005). Do you remember? How caregivers question their spouses who have Alzheimer's disease and the impact on communication. *Journal of Speech, Language, and Hearing Research, 48*, 125–136.

Tappen, R., Williams-Burgess, C., Edelstein, J., Touhy, T., & Fishman, S. (1997). Communicating with individuals with Alzheimer's disease: Examination of recommended strategies. *Archives of Psychiatric Nursing, 11*(5), 249–256.

Turkstra, L., & Bourgeois, M. (2005). Interventions for a modern day HM: Errorless learning of practical goals. *Journal of Medical Speech-Language Pathology, 13*, 205–212.

Vanderslott, J. (1994). A positive exercise in damage limitation: Management of aggression in elderly confused people. *Professional Nurse, 10*(3), 150–152.

PART

Additional Considerations in Treatment of Dementia

The third part of this book addresses other aspects of dementia treatment and important external factors that play a part in the care of your patients, family members, and caregivers. Chapter 10 gives ideas and advice on approaching patient and family education and training with some helpful educational handouts on common dementia-related topics. Chapter 11 deals with the topic of documentation and reimbursement. Chapter 12 addresses some of the behavioral issues that commonly are associated with many of the dementia diagnoses that we deal with frequently. Chapter 13 gives a brief summary of some of the pharmacological and non-pharmacological intervention available for your patients. Chapter 14 is about the team approach and the importance of taking a holistic approach when treating patients with dementia. The final chapter provides some special considerations for the home health therapist in providing some extra information and resources to those clinicians who are working with patients in the community.

10

Counseling, Teaching, and Supporting

Introduction

There is more to what we do than only assessment, goal planning, and therapeutic intervention with the dementia population. We have not completed our job until we have incorporated some education, teaching and/or counseling with the family, caregiver, and quite possibly the patient themselves. Why is this so important that it deserves its own chapter? Because, at the end of the day, when you are ready to discharge your patient from service, they still will have dementia; it is not going away. We are obligated to help the patient and family prepare for the road ahead by giving them the knowledge and resources that are necessary to cope and make appropriate healthcare decisions in the future, as well as help them cope with the difficult situations they face daily. This chapter will offer some guidance in counseling and educating and offer some handouts and resources that may be helpful to you in your practice.

Understanding Grief

Your interactions with patients and family members dealing with dementia will be varied and unpredictable. The reason being that each individual experiences trauma, illness, and loss differently. Because the diagnosis of dementia is considered terminal and means the certain loss of memory, personality, and eventually life, it is likely that family members will go through a grieving process while their loved one still is living. The patients themselves also may be experiencing the grieving process, which may manifest itself in behaviors and reactions toward you or their family members.

The Five Stages of Grief

Elizabeth Kubler-Ross was a psychiatrist who studied the effects of grief on human beings. She was able to develop a framework and a set of tools for people to use to help identify the process of grief. The five stages of grief are common landmarks of behavior or thought processes that people generally experience when grieving. The stages are not always experienced sequentially or in any specific time frame. Understanding the stages of grief may help you understand the emotions, reactions, and behaviors of the loved ones you work to council and educate. The following is a summary of information about the five stages taken from Dr. Kubler-Ross's book titled *On Death and Dying* (Kubler-Ross, 1969).

Denial

Denial and shock are coping mechanisms that help people deal with the situation. A family member or even the patient may be in the denial stage for a long time after learning about the diagnosis of dementia. You may hear phrases such as, "I want to get a second opinion" or "my mother never had a good memory anyway" and "we are going to beat this!" The act of denial is not defiant in nature but a way for the mind to protect the individual from being immersed in the tragedy and reality of the diagnosis. Dealing with family who are working through denial may be tough for an SLP as there may be a great deal of resistance to treatment ideas (i.e., not wanting to put labels or signs up that are reminders of the disease), or they may want any and all intervention available because there are some unreal expectations.

The best advice we can give is to be compassionate and understanding that denial is part of the process of acceptance and your approach is to acknowledge and validate feelings while at the same time be realistic. It is not necessary to "sugar coat" the situation and, at the same time, it is not appropriate to force the harsh reality of dementia upon the family or that patient and squashing any hope of quality of life. Find a balance in your approach and in time this stage may pass—in some instances, it may not be until the end of life.

Anger

Once the realization is made that denial is not an option, the next stage is anger. This can manifest itself in many different ways, and the therapist or medical personnel frequently are the target of that anger. It is important for the SLP to stay detached and not take any attacks personally. Occasionally, the family members of the demented take their anger out on their loved one with the disease. It is not uncommon to see the children become overtly disgusted and impatient with behaviors or during interactions with their parents. The SLP can use gentle suggestions for better communication strategies and for anger outlets for the family member suffering through the anger stage. For patients who may be suffering through this stage, using de-escalation techniques as well as validation strategies can help subdue an angry situation.

Bargaining

At this stage we may see family members desperately looking for a cure or magic fix for the dementia. They may see progress toward a goal when the therapist sees very little progress and needs to discharge from therapy. This is the stage where the family member will refuse to put their loved one on hospice in lieu of trying speech therapy or medication alteration. The best approach in this stage is to be a good listener and mirror what is being said. It does little help to argue or try to convince somebody that there is "no hope." If the case presents itself that the family member is looking for speech therapy when you as the therapist do not see it as a viable option (meaning that it is your opinion that the patient will not be able to effectively participate or meet goals), then you need to present facts to justify your decision. These facts may include objective scores from a screening tool, which illustrates the patient's inability to follow instructions or actively participate.

Depression

Depression can occur at any stage of the process. At this stage of grieving, it is common to see increased tearfulness of the family member. It is very difficult to see a loved one deteriorate and just as horrifying not to be recognizable by your own husband, wife, or mother. Your job is to be compassionate, listen, and provide support to the loved one. During this time in the grieving process, it is common for loved ones to be less visible. Visits are fewer and far between. Sometimes absence is one of the ways for the loved one to work through this stage of grief. Our job is not to diagnose or offer treatment for any patient or family member who is depressed. However, we can use our knowledge of the signs and symptoms of depression to understand behaviors and to interact with compassion and understanding of this process of grieving.

Acceptance

Accepting the reality of the dementia can bring forth a number of ethical challenges for the SLP. Realization of what the future holds may be the catalyst for family members to discontinue therapy services. Realizing that there is no cure for the dementia, the family member may decide to ask the physician to discontinue dementia medications. There is no right or wrong in this decision process, however, many family members are not prepared for the sudden rapid decline in functioning that can occur after discontinuing medications. This decline cannot be reversed after the medication is stopped.

Family members also may decide to allow loved ones freedom to discontinue swallow precautions or dietary regimens. These decisions usually are made with well-meaning intentions but can pose additional health and safety risks to the patient. It is our job to ensure that the family members are very well informed and educated regarding the consequence of their decisions. We should do this in an objective manner and not in a way that displays our bias toward the situation.

Frequently during the acceptance phase, the family member can become more relaxed around their loved one. We often see less arguing or correcting and more nurturing and understanding. It often is as if the battle to accept is over and a sense of calm develops in the relationship. At this point, family members often acquiesce to enlisting hospice services, which usually means it is time for the speech therapist to exit the scene (as therapy services generally are not covered when a patient is under hospice care).

The Approach

You are preparing to educate a family member of your patient who has dementia. You have gathered all kinds of brochures, handouts, and videos designed to help the family member deal with their demented loved one. Before you open up your PowerPoint presentation, take a moment to step back and look at the person you are educating. It is likely that they are simultaneously dealing with at least 50 other issues surrounding their loved one's care, not to mention likely dealing with some fatigue and illness of their own. There are daily stresses that we cannot even imagine, not to mention the sadness of watching their loved one become someone they no longer recognize. So, if you were to throw an armload of information at this family member, they are likely to retain the information only until you walk out the door and they have to return to being the caregiver. The following is a list of suggested approaches to education and training.

Start Immediately

Do not wait until the end of your Plan of Care and the day of discharge to unload information on the caregiver. Start at the very beginning. Educate as topics arise and allow the family member time to come up with questions or concerns. Make it a point to begin each session with a follow-up question from the last session, such as "In the last session, we talked about the chin tuck swallow strategy. Do you feel comfortable with this information? Did you think of any questions you would like to ask me about that strategy?" The follow-up question allows you to present the information a second time and gives you the opportunity to gauge the learning level of your audience. If you are having to re-educate each time you present the follow-up question, a different approach may be necessary.

A Little at a Time

Give only a little information at a time. Do not overwhelm the already overwhelmed family member with several topics of information all at once. It is helpful to plan ahead of time for a short education/information session for each visit. This can be done by using a calendar and selecting a topic for each visit day. Use this as a check-off list as you progress through the calendar. Offer no more than two handouts of information at a time during an information session.

Keep It Simple

Short, sweet, and to the point. Use simple handouts that are bulleted, written in lay terms, and easy to read. Make sure the caregiver has time to look over the information and take notes as you discuss each topic. If possible, offer the caregiver a folder to keep therapy-related information and education materials. Encourage the caregiver to write down questions inbetween therapy sessions as they arise.

Allow Time

Try to build time into your sessions to allow for education and training so that you do not have to rush through it because you have another patient to see. At the same time, be mindful of family members or caregivers that may dominate your session with questions. Let them know that you have set aside 10 minutes at the end of the session for education/discussion. Stick to your timetable and have the family member write down any questions you did not get to address for the next session.

Education for the Patient

The patient should be included as much as possible during the education process. Never assume that the patient will not benefit from education despite the diagnosis. Even if the patient does not understand the content or implications of the education, sometimes it makes them feel as though they have a little more control of the situation and their own care, which is very rare for the dementia patient. If the subject matter is sensitive and needs to be discussed with a family member (i.e., discussing behavior issues), then it would be prudent to schedule a time outside of the therapy session to provide education and discussion. It can be awkward to leave the room with the caregiver or family member leaving the patient behind while you have a discussion. Therefore, it is best to plan in advance with the family member a time to meet to provide information and training. Make it a point to telephone or email the family member the day before to let them know that you need to find time for a private discussion outside of the regularly scheduled therapy time.

Documentation

It is very important that each time you offer education, training, or in-servicing of facility staff that it is well documented. Education and training is a necessary and expected component of treatment, and you should make sure that you are credited for doing your job. At the same time, it always is good to have documented evidence of education in the event that an incidence occurs and the family member claims they were not properly educated.

Counseling

It is well within the scope of practice for the SLP to provide ongoing counseling and support throughout the therapy process. Of course, the SLP is not working toward solving any major issues with the patient or family member, but merely being available as a sounding board and to offer support when needed. Oftentimes, the therapist is able to draw from a multitude of past experiences with other patients in order to counsel and offer support. Frequently, the family member who is in the caregiver role is looking for someone to listen, as there may be minimal opportunities for the family member to talk with adults outside of their own loved one whom they are caring for. It is important to follow a few basic rules when providing counseling during your therapy session.

1. Keep your comments to a minimum. You may be more effective as a sounding board rather than offering advice or lengthy explanations. Frequently the caregiver is able to solve their own riddles just by listening to you paraphrase what already has been said. Refrain from adding your own anecdotes or personal family stories into the conversation. This can alter the client/clinician relationship by allowing the client to become personally involved in the clinician's business.

2. Validate. Even if you completely disagree with the issue or the message from the caregiver (or the patient for that matter), it is best to validate what is being said. It can be very helpful for a frustrated caregiver to hear the clinician validate his/her feelings and emotions.

3. Take it outside. It is easy to start chatting about the patient while the patient still is present (especially during the later stages of the disease). Get into the habit early on of assuming that the patient knows and understands every word that is being said (and likely does!). Always discuss sensitive issues away from the patient or actively include the patient in the conversation. It may sound like this: "Mr. Hale, I hope you don't mind if I have a conversation with your wife. I promise that we are not ignoring you!"

4. Watch your time! Although counseling indeed is a very important part of our jobs, it also can become a time sucker. It is very important to be mindful of your time and is important to be prudent with the time spent providing service to your patient. Family members can easily become very verbose when sharing their frustrations and emotions of loss and grief. It is helpful when beginning a conversation with a family member by being inviting yet also setting limits. For example, the conversation can be initiated like this:

   "Please tell me about your frustrating night last night . . . I have five minutes before I have to leave for my next appointment." This introduction sets limits immediately so that the clinician will not have to feel uncomfortable when he/she has to interrupt the caregiver to remind him/her of your need to leave the conversation.

5. Offer resources. You can be most helpful to the caregiver by redirecting them to outside resources. This might include an Alzheimer's support group in their area or professional counselors or psychologists who can spend more quality time working, listening, and helping with emotional issues that occur with caregivers.

6. Do not try to fix it. Dementia is a destroyer of many things besides just a person's memories. It affects relationships and the health and well-being of the caregiver. You will not be able to fix all of the problems that come along

with a diagnosis of dementia. But BEWARE! If you are able to fix one problem, like a swallowing deficit, family members may be latching onto you to fix a multitude of other problems as well. It is important to be able to distance yourself enough to say "no" and to redirect. It is very easy to get pulled into the drama of someone else's family or relationship and difficult to know when to pull back and step away.

Take Care of Yourself

The authors of this book frequently are asked, "How do you deal with working with such a depressing group of people?" This question is commonly followed by "Don't you get depressed?" Our response is generally "no." We feel a great sense of gratification in working with this population and definitely feel we are making a difference in the lives of the dementia patient and family members. That is not to say that there are not days when we feel emotionally drained, especially if we are doing a great deal of counseling and supporting. It is important to be able to identify in yourself the signs of stress that may be a result of the job. If you suspect that you are beginning to feel sad, overwhelmed, and/or overly frustrated with your patients or family members, understand that it is okay to back away and allow a colleague to step in for a while. If you can, seek some other clients who do not have dementia in order to give yourself a break. You may need to set the reset button in order to find more success and energy to deal with your patients.

Summary

Counseling, giving guidance, providing feedback, and education is likely the most important aspect of the SLP's job when working with dementia. Although you may not be able to say, "I've been there" when you are listening to your patient or caregiver work through issues of anger or acceptance, you will be able to say "I understand and I am here to help," which can be very comforting and soothing. The education and counseling you are able to provide will help positively impact the patient and family member long after your therapy session ends.

Reference

Kubler-Ross, E. (1969). *On death and dying.* New York, NY: Touchstone.

11

Documentation: Connecting the Dots

Introduction

You now are finding that you are much more empowered with your dementia patients. Your assessment skills, planning, and treatment execution are proving to be very successful, and your patients are making progress. However, if you do not accurately document what you have accomplished (or even attempted but *not* accomplished), you will not be paid for all of the time and effort you have spent with your patients. Good documentation is extremely important, as always, but at this time in history when the government is scrutinizing every dime spent on health care, accurate, efficient, and sufficient documentation is more important than ever.

According to the American Speech-Language-Hearing Association, the SLP's documentation should include findings of the speech-language evaluation, objective/subjective measurements of functioning, short-term and long-term measurement of goals, as well as the expectations for progress, frequency of service, and a reasonable estimate of duration of service. ASHA further states that claims for our services must be supported through our documentation that should illustrate the following:

1. Reasonable: Treatment is given in the appropriate amount, at the appropriate frequency and duration in accordance with accepted standards of practice.

2. Necessary: Treatment is appropriate for the patient's diagnosis and condition.

3. Specific: Treatment is targeted toward particular treatment goals.

4. Effective: Treatment is expected to yield improvement within a reasonable time.

5. Skilled: The treatment provided required the complex skills, knowledge, and judgment of a SLP (American Speech-Language-Hearing Association, 2011).

In working with the dementia population, it often is good practice to ask yourself each time you document "Is this reasonable, necessary, specific, effective, and skilled?" If you answer "no" to any of the above, or have doubt or hesitation, it may be time to rethink your actions. Many clinicians become complacent with documentation. Our writing has become automatic and robotic not only as a method of time efficiency but also as a matter of habit. We develop documentation habits because we are stuck in a documentation "rut." All of the elements provided by the ASHA above are important, but ensuring that your treatment focus and documentation is specific to one patient in particular will allow you to stay clear from developing poor documentation patterns.

Why Do We Have to Document?

A good place to start is behind the question "Why do we need to document?" It sounds rather obvious, but there is more than one answer to this question beyond "because we need to show what we did in therapy." The World Health Organization (WHO) is the directing and coordinating authority for health within the United Nations system. It consists of 8,000 public health experts responsible for providing leadership on global health matters, shaping health research, setting standards, and monitoring health trends. WHO is a good source to turn to for guidelines and trends in documentation.

WHO would answer that there are multiple reasons for good documentation, including communication between professionals, accountability to their professional practice, legislative requirements, and quality improvement. Your documentation serves as a link between the patient, other healthcare professionals, and fiscal intermediaries (World Health Organization, 2007). Furthermore, what you put down on paper may serve as a tool for treatment planning for this patient and others like them in the future.

There is no magic formula for documenting your interventions with the dementia patient. The same clear, concise, documentation that you provide for all of your other patients applies. Let us take a look at the basics required for documentation and then see how that can apply to your cognitively challenged patients. WHO has set forth some basic documentation guidelines that we have adopted to help you understand what is needed in your documentation. We have added to these guidelines to make them more pertinent to documenting for dementia.

The Who, What, When, Why, and How of Dementia Documentation

Who?

Documentation is a record of your first-hand knowledge, observation, actions, decisions, and outcomes. It is an official record of skilled intervention by a skilled professional. Of course it is important to document not only who you are but also who else is involved in this patient's care (i.e., caregivers, family members, other therapists, medical social worker).

What?

This relates to what is happening with the patient and includes all subjective and objective information, including observations, assessments, actions, outcomes, and variances from outcomes. This information is important in building the rationale for your intervention. For instance, in working with a demented patient living at home with his wife, it is important to document "what" the patient was doing prior to your involvement (i.e., Patient was wandering outside into busy intersection), "what" the patient was doing during your therapy (i.e., Patient participating in Spaced Retrieval techniques to learn how to exit the house safely), and "what" the patient was doing after your intervention (i.e., Patient no longer exits into the busy street. Patient uses back door exit to secure backyard).

When?

This is a record of when therapy or events took place. This includes critical incidents (i.e., falls, illness) in addition to therapeutic events. The "when" of documentation is important in working with dementia patients as measures of performance and behaviors in therapy often can be dictated by the time of day (i.e., sundowning behaviors). Having an accurate account of events during a time of the day/week can become very useful for other health-care professionals. As an example, the dementia patient is presenting with a change in participation with increased fatigue, agitation, and frustration during the speech therapy visits. Review of the documentation reveals that the physical therapist, who visits in the mornings has increased the exercise regimen, incorporating walking outside. Consequently, the patient is exhausted in the afternoons by the time the SLP comes to perform treatment. Documentation should illustrate a natural time line of events so that there is no question to the reviewer of when therapy or events occurred.

Why?

The "why" is likely the most important aspect of clinical documentation. This is the basis of communication between healthcare professionals and is used to demonstrate accountability. Why are you working with the patient? Of course the easiest answer is 'because they are in need of skilled speech-language pathology services' and there is no better answer than that. However, the SLP always should justify intervention by explaining why there is a need to provide services. In documenting for dementia therapy, this can be easily explained in conjunction with the "What" from above. The patient, who is wandering out into the busy street needs skilled speech therapy intervention . . . WHY? Because he is at risk for accidental injury. Documentation on an assessment may look like this:

> " . . . skilled speech-language pathology intervention is indicated as patient's wandering behaviors put him at great risk for accidental injury to self."

How?

WHO puts the "how" into a very simple approach. Documentation must be clear, concise, and true. It must be legible and permanent, current, confidential, and chronological. Documentation must be based on observations and assessment, consistent with guidelines and legislation and avoid ambiguity (World Health Organization, 2007). The "how" is the complete package. Documentation must tell a complete story to somebody who may not even have any understanding of what a SLP does, or what the effects of dysphagia can have on the patient with dementia. If all of the "How" is incorporated in the documentation, there will be little room for question, doubt, or denial.

A Quick Word About Denials

Many clinicians are under the impression that treatment of patients with dementia leads to automatic denials from insurance companies and Medicare intermediaries. The fact is that many intermediaries will pay for therapy provided to a patient with dementia providing there is adequate documentation that reflects the treatment was medically indicated and there was progress toward stated (realistic) goals. The Department of Health and Human Services (DHHS) and the Centers for Medicare and Medicaid Services (CMS) broadcast *Transmittal AB-01-135* on September 25, 2001. This transmittal stated, "Contractors may not install edits that result in the automatic denial of services based solely on the ICD-9 codes for dementia" (Department of Health and Human Services, 2001). This transmittal further states that people with dementia indeed may benefit from speech-language pathology and other therapies. CMS cautions us that dementia "may not support the medical necessity of a Medicare benefit when covered alone" (Department of Health and Human Services, 2001), instructing us to use secondary diagnoses or conditions as well as the diagnosis of dementia. It should be understood that although having the proper diagnosis on your documentation is important, it does not guarantee that Medicare indeed will accept this patient's claim. The important part of the claim is how well the treatment or assessment was communicated (see "Who, What, When, and How" above).

Show Me the Data!

In some cases, it appears that our colleagues in physical therapy have life a little easier when it comes to demonstrating progress. It is much easier to quantify progress with grip strength, gait speed, and range of motion using tools of measurement. The progress of a cognitively impaired person may not be so clearly visible or as easily quantifiable as overt signs and appearances may have little or no variance. This is why the use of data collection is very important in documentation.

Although it is not practical to perform a standardized assessment to measure progress during each and every visit with a demented patient, it is important to collect and record data. This does not have to be labor intensive or exhaustive. In fact, the simpler the data collection, the easier it is to illustrate progress or decline.

Keep in mind that something of value has to be recorded with each visit. That value can be a positive or a negative value (depending on the progress of the patient). Some examples may include:

1. Patient was able to demonstrate an increase in recalling his safety cue for exiting to 5 minutes from initial cue. (An increase in 2 minutes from last session.)

2. Patient was able to demonstrate his chin tuck during meal eight out of 10 times (80%) using a Spaced Retrieval cue. (An increase of 20% from last visit.)

3. Patient was able to communicate basic need (I am thirsty) using gestural communication when prompted five out of 10 trials. (An increase of 10% from last visit.)

4. Patient recalled his room number three out of 10 trials using Spaced Retrieval prompt. (A decrease of 20% from last visit.)

5. Patient scored a 15 out of 30 on the SLUMS evaluation. (An increase of five points from initial evaluation performed on 10/5/12.)

It also is important to illustrate to the reader how the performance during a single therapy task is functional and reasonable. For instance, if you are documenting that a patient is recalling his safety cue to extinguish exit seeking, it is helpful to have a statement as to how this improves his functioning by decreasing his risk for accidental injury. You may go even further to express (in your subjective documentation section) that the patient's wife reported that patient is recalling his strategies with increased frequency, reducing anxiety behaviors that usually are present when the wife has to keep him from leaving the house.

Get Out of Your Rut

For many of us who have been working as clinicians throughout the decades, documentation becomes second nature. We have templates of terminology, phrases, and paragraphs that have served us in the past and used so much that they flow automatically and effortlessly into the medical record. Therapists often become very comfortable in using these repeated patterns as if stuck in a rut. This rut is a dangerous place to be with regard to documentation as the clinician easily strays from creating a document that is specific and individualized to each patient. We are fortunate to be moving into the age of electronic medical record keeping, which has proven to be more efficient, time saving, and economical for health care professionals. However, the "cut and paste" functions of our keyboards in fact may be our worst enemy.

There are some common words/phrases/terminology that are commonly used by SLPs that do not provide any content or meaning to the medical record when used independently.

We have chosen a few to illustrate how using detail specific to the patient can improve the integrity of the documentation.

Continue Plan of Care

Although it is important to state that you are or are not going to continue with the treatment plan that was stated during the evaluation process, it is very important each time to document "what" it is you plan to do on your next visit. Providing a clear statement of what your intention is for the next therapy visit lets the reviewer know that you are following an organized Plan of Care, using your skilled clinical knowledge and expertise to successfully guide this patient to meeting his/her goals. Now of course, we all know that with the unpredictable nature of the dementia population, the plan may not be followed exactly as written from the previous visit. As long as it is documented as to why that plan was altered, there should be no question as to the decision-making process. Here are some good documentation examples:

> "Will continue working with patient on environmental orientation using landmark identification. Will specifically work on helping patient locate facility dining room to increase independence and reduce signs/symptoms of anxiety exhibited prior to meals."

> "Will add goals to treatment plan for communication of basic needs during meal time as facility staff have reported patient demonstrating anxiety while trying to communicate entrée choices from menu."

> "Continue working on long-term goal for safe swallow using the Spaced Retrieval technique. Will begin educating patient's wife on using SR cues for chin tuck."

Patient Alert and Oriented

It is doubtful that our dementia patients really are oriented unless they are using an external device or cueing system. However, perhaps they really are alert and oriented—in that case, it is *very* important to justify why you are working with them. It is recommended that this "alert and oriented" be used sparingly or expanded to more detail:

> "Patient was attentive during our therapy session today with little or no redirection to task required."

> "Patient was oriented to self only. He reported that he returned home from his honeymoon yesterday and was searching for his wife. This therapist validated his feelings of excitement and concern during therapy in order to reduce his anxiety. Patient was easily redirected to therapy tasks following validation approach."

No Progress

It is true that there are clinicians out there who will document "no progress" and yet continue to treat their patients. It should be no surprise that a claim might be denied after multiple entries of "no progress" were noted in the documentation. Continuing to treat a patient when progress toward goals is not evident is problematic . This little phrase also should be used very sparingly, perhaps only on the two entries of documentation. If the term "red flag" should be used any time in this manual, this is the time to use it! "No progress" means that the patient is not moving forward with the stated plan and either needs to discharge or the plan should be altered. So, if you are going to use this terminology and continue with treatment, it is necessary to expand:

> "Patient has not demonstrated progress toward his long-term goal of using chin tuck independently for safe swallow of thin liquids. Will implement new long-term goal of safe swallow with thickened liquids."

> "Patient has not demonstrated progress with word-finding goals during this session. Patient had been demonstrating steady progress in therapy up until this date. Poor progress today is likely secondary to patient recovering from upper respiratory infection. Will attempt the same goal next visit before altering the Plan of Care."

> "Patient has not been able to demonstrate progress toward long- or short-term goals during the past two visits. Met with patient's physician, who reports patient has demonstrated an overall decline in health due to secondary dehydration. Will hold speech therapy services for one week per physician request and resume therapy upon physician recommendation."

Added Enhancements

There are some words and phrases that may be beneficial to your documentation to indicate that your treatment is reasonable and necessary. This terminology puts a positive light on the therapeutic process and sets a tone for a positive clinical expectation:

> "Patient is highly motivated."

> "Patient's wife has been educated on safe swallow strategies and completed return demonstration without assistance."

> "Patient is compliant with current diet restrictions."

> "Prognosis for meeting goals is good."

Conclusion

A colleague once gave a lecture on documentation presenting two pieces of artwork. The first piece of artwork was obviously drawn by a small child with two-dimensional stick figures and crudely placed shapes that had us guessing it was a landscape with a tree and a house. The second piece of artwork was a beautiful landscape painted by a well-known artist. The colors and textures were rich and detailed, leaving no question as to the content. It was evident from the use of colors and the detail of the content that the landscape was depicting the fall season. The painting was so realistic that the viewer was immediately transported to that place and time. My colleague asked the audience the question "which piece of artwork is representative of your documentation?" The point being that we are supposed to be painting a picture with our words so that there is no room for error in our interpretation. Treatment of the dementia population does not require any more documentation than our treatment of cognitively intact patients. We need to make sure we are painting a clear picture for those who may not understand what we do, who we do it for, and why we do what we do.

References

American Speech-Language-Hearing Association (ASHA). (2011). *Speech-language pathology medical review guidelines.* Retrieved April 20, 2013, from http://www.asha.org

Department of Health and Human Services (DHHS). (2001, September 25). *Program Memorandum; Intermediaries/carriers; transmittal AB-01-135.* Centers for Medicare and Medicaid Services (CMS). CMS-Pub, 60AB.

World Health Organization (WHO). (2007). Guidelines for medial record and clinical documentation. *WHO-SEARO Coding Workshop* (pp. 1–16). Author.

12

Behavioral Issues

*Many people find the changes in behavior caused by Alzheimer's to be
the most challenging and distressing effect of the disease.*

(Alzheimer's Association, 2013a)

The behavioral symptoms associated with dementia often are difficult to understand and
treat for both the skilled professional and the patient's caregivers and loved ones. This
chapter will explore the most common behavioral symptoms related to dementia and
provide a framework for analyzing challenging behaviors in order to better understand
and manage them.

Common Behavioral Symptoms Associated With Dementia

During the early stages of dementia, the presence of behavioral symptoms may reveal
themselves through changes in personality, such as anxiety, irritability, and/or depression
(Alzheimer's Association, 2013a). As dementia progresses, these behavioral symptoms
may progress or additional symptoms may arise such as anger, agitation, aggression,
emotional distress, changes in sleep, and verbal and physical outbursts (Alzheimer's Association, 2013a). These symptoms may result in challenging behaviors such as wandering,
repetitive question asking, decreased appetite or intake, repetitive motions or vocalizations, or socially inappropriate behavior. As with any of the common characteristics of
dementia, the presence of these symptoms can be highly individualized, resulting in
patients who display a number of behavioral challenges or very few of them. It is important for the professional working with the dementia population to be aware of these
symptoms to assist caregivers in understanding and dealing with these changes, as well
as to participate in the treatment and management of these challenges.

So how do these behavioral symptoms manifest themselves into challenging caregiving situations? Below are some common scenarios that may occur in a facility or home setting. We use some of these examples as a framework to better understand and treat behavioral challenges throughout the remainder of this chapter.

- A nursing home resident requests assistance from facility staff to use the restroom several times a day, even after he recently has visited the restroom.
- A woman living at home begins to ask her husband the same questions over and over again several times a day and seems unsatisfied with the responses that her husband provides.
- An assisted-living patient begins to refuse to leave his apartment for activities and meals and becomes anxious and angry when staff and family try to encourage him to participate in these activities.
- A nursing home patient begins to eat less and less at meals and becomes very aggressive with staff and other residents sitting at his dining table, causing distress for the patient, the other residents, and the staff trying to assist the patient.
- A participant at an adult day program constantly tries to leave the building or is found wandering in unsafe areas throughout the day.
- A nursing home patient refuses to participate in bathing with the facility staff and often becomes verbally and physically aggressive to staff throughout the process.
- A sub-acute patient recovering from hip replacement surgery frequently is trying to get out of bed without assistance, increasing his risk of falling and/or additional injury.
- A man who recently moved in with his daughter and her family frequently forgets to take his medications throughout the day while he is home alone and repeatedly asks his daughter when he is going to be able to go back to living in his own home.

Understanding Behavioral Symptoms

The behavioral and personality changes associated with dementia can be difficult to understand. In order to understand these changes, it is important to first examine why they occur. The leading cause for these symptoms is the changes occurring in the brain due to the presence of a disease, such as Alzheimer's, and its overall effects on the processes of the brain. However, there may be other reasons/causes for the presence of these symptoms that should be examined, such as medication, environmental influences/changes, and the presence of additional medical conditions (Alzheimer's Association, 2013a).

According to the Family Caregiver Alliance, it is important to first remember that behavior has a purpose (Family Caregiver Alliance, 2013). The behaviors that may be considered to be problematic or challenging for us as the patient's caregivers actually are a form of communication for the person with dementia. By looking at behavior as a form of communication, we can try to better understand why it is occurring. Asking questions such as, "What is the person trying to tell us by acting or not acting a certain way?"; "What purpose is the behavior serving to the person with dementia?"; and "Why is this behavior occurring (in this environment, at this time of day, in this situation, etc.)?" can assist in better understanding behavioral challenges in dementia.

Researcher Jiska Cohen-Mansfield and her colleagues are leaders in understanding behavior and agitation in persons with dementia. Their research states that, "most agitated behaviors are manifestations of unmet needs (of the patient)" (Camp, Cohen-Mansfield, & Capezuti, 2002, p. 1397). These unmet needs may be related to areas such as physiologic issues (undiagnosed/untreated pain), safety (fear of being hurt), love and belonging (fear of being abandoned), and self-actualization (lack of meaningful role within one's life or environment). "The effects of dementia leave the (person with dementia) unable to fulfill these needs because of a combination of perceptual problems, communication difficulties, and an inability to manipulate the environment through appropriate channels" (Camp et al., 2002, p. 1397). See Table 12–1 for a listing of possible unmet needs and behaviors based on Cohen-Mansfield's findings. Analyzing behaviors using the framework of unmet needs can be used in both home and facility settings in

Table 12–1. Analyzing Possible Unmet Needs and Possible Related Behavioral Challenges for Persons With Dementia

Unmet Need	Description	Possible Related Behaviors
Physiologic	Undiagnosed/Untreated pain or illness (e.g., urinary tract infection, other infection/illness, neuropathy, etc.)	Aggression Agitation Increased memory loss Personality changes
Safety	Fear of being hurt; Feeling unsafe in environment	Combativeness Verbal aggression Wandering/Elopement
Love and Belonging	Fear of being abandoned (e.g., fear of not seeing loved ones)	Wandering Elopement Repetitive question asking of where loved ones are, when they are visiting, etc. Repeatedly asking to go home
Self-Actualization	Having a meaningful role within one's environment; Engaging in meaningful activity	Wandering Excessive sleeping Refusal to participate in activities Repetitive question asking

order to determine what purpose the behavior is serving for the person with dementia and thereby can lead to the development of more effective treatment options to reduce the likelihood of the behavior occurring.

It also is important to note that we as caregivers have more control over modifying our own behavior than we do in modifying the behavior of the person with dementia (Family Caregiver Alliance, 2013). Using strategies such as reducing the length and complexity of our speech, breaking down tasks into simple, repeatable steps, and listening to the patient can help to modify the persons behavior by making the information we are sharing with them easier to understand.

Analyzing Behavioral Symptoms

Understanding why a behavior is occurring is the first step in developing possible treatment solutions. Once you have examined the patient's possible unmet needs as possible reasons for the behavior, you also may need to do further analysis related to areas such as:

1. The patient's environment.

2. The patient's daily routine (or lack thereof).

3. Personal causes such as a need for attention, reassurance, social interaction, and so forth.

4. The patient's own opinion/communication related to the behavior.

5. Strategies that have been both successful and unsuccessful to alleviate/reduce the behavior thus far.

6. Answering the questions "Is the problem really a problem?" and "Who owns the problem?" (i.e., "Is the problem more of a problem to others and not to the patient himself?" For example, if the patient constantly mismatches their clothing, is this more of a problem for the patient's family in accepting how the patient looks and less to the patient who still is trying to dress themselves?)

To best examine behavioral challenges, we recommend developing a "Brainstorm Session" with other professionals who are working with the client and/or the patient's family in order to best define why a behavior is occurring. If it is not possible to have a meeting to discuss these issues, we recommend brainstorming yourself all possible reasons that the behavior may serve as well as possible triggers that may be leading to the exhibiting of the behavior. This may involve observing the patient for a period of time and recording when the behavior occurs in order to determine if there is a pattern or a trigger causing the behavior.

For example, using the first scenario presented in this chapter, if a nursing facility patient is regularly requesting assistance to use the restroom after just having visited the restroom, it would be beneficial to observe the time of day this typically occurs, what is he doing (or not doing) at that time, and so forth, in order to determine possible reasons for the behavior. It may be that he typically asks for this assistance at times during the day when there is little to no activity occurring in the facility and therefore he seeks out the social contact of a staff member to assist him in the restroom (**unmet need: self-actualization/lack of meaningful engagement**). It also could be that a change in medication has caused him to feel like he needs to use the restroom more often (**unmet need: physiologic change**) or that he is forgetting he just has used the restroom altogether (**short term memory loss related to physiologic changes in brain**). All three of these possible reasons for the patient's repetitive requests to use the restroom would have different treatment solutions. If the patient is seeking social interaction through this behavior, providing him with a written checklist of when he last visited the restroom would not decrease the occurrence of the behavior, but if the reason he requests bathroom visits frequently is because he cannot remember the last time he was there, a checklist might be useful in reducing this behavior. Therefore, it is important to first understand the root or cause of the behavior in order to develop related and successful treatment solutions.

Figure 12–1 is a worksheet that can be used to help "brainstorm" possible reasons for behavioral symptoms. At the end of this chapter, you will find completed "Behavior Brainstorming Worksheets" for the scenarios presented at the beginning of this chapter to further serve as examples.

Developing Treatment Solutions for Behavioral Challenges

We now explore how to develop possible solutions for some selected behavioral problems. We would like to emphasize that the treatment solutions listed here are not extensive and may not work for every patient. It is important to first discover why the person is exhibiting the behavior and then choose solutions that best fit these reasons. This may result in some "trial and error" of different solutions before one that works is discovered. Over time, it may be found that a solution that once alleviated a behavior no longer works. This may be due to a change in the individual related to the progression of dementia or another medical need arising or another behavior replacing the one that was eliminated. In any case, the team working with the patient should return to brainstorming possible reasons and solutions and remain flexible to the changing needs of the patient.

It should be noted that a skilled rehabilitation professional, such as a speech-language pathologist (SLP), can be an integral part of the process of understanding and treating behavioral issues with persons with dementia. The process of understanding behavior is highly skilled, and the development and implementation of interventions can be a billable and reimbursable service for rehabilitation. As discussed extensively in Chapter 8, it is important that goals addressing behavioral symptoms be written explicitly to demonstrate the behavior(s) being targeted, why the behavior is being addressed, the treatment method that will be utilized, and include a criterion to measure progress. It also is important that nursing staff and/or other treating professionals regularly document the presence of the behavior and the behavior's overall effects on the patients health and

Behavior Brainstorming Worksheet

Patient: _____

Challenging Behavior: _____

Possible Reasons for Behavior (list all possible ideas):

_____

_____

_____

_____

_____

_____

_____

Possible Unmet Needs (circle any applicable & list why):

Physiologic _____   Love & Belonging _____

Safety   _____   Self-Actualization _____

Possible Contributory Factors (circle all that apply):

Environment   Need for Reassurance   Other_____
Routine (or lack of)   Need for Social Interaction   _____
Need for Attention   Other Residents/Triggers   _____

Times When Behavior Typically Occurs ("Is there a pattern?") _____

_____

Times When Behavior Is Not Occurring _____

_____

Patient Aware of Behavior? Y / N

Patient's Response to Questions About Behavior: _____

_____

Previous Responses/Strategies to Reduce Behavior: _____

_____

Possible New Strategies to Try to Reduce Behavior (list staff responsible for implementation & date to reassess):

_____

_____

_____

_____

_____

Rehabilitation Referral Needed: Y / N (PT   OT   SLP)
Name of Staff Obtaining Referral:

Figure 12–1. Behavior brainstorming worksheet.

safety in order to provide support for the patient to be seen by a rehabilitation professional for the issue. After discussion of each of the following behavioral challenges, you
will find an example of a goal(s) that may be utilized by the SLP to address the issue
during skilled treatment.

Behavioral Challenge: Wandering

The term "wandering" is used to describe the behavior of seemingly moving aimlessly
about one's environment. The Alzheimer's Association reports that one in six persons
with dementia will wander (Alzheimer's Association, 2013b). The term wandering implies
that the person has no purpose in their movement, when in fact the act of wandering
is likely fulfilling a need for him/her. That need could be the need for movement, the
fact that they are seeking out something, such as food or social interaction, or that they
simply are bored and need to be engaged in something more interesting. Wandering can
lead to safety risks such as falling, walking into unsafe areas that could result in injury,
getting lost or leaving one's home or facility environment unattended. It is important to
first discover what need wandering is fulfilling for the patient in order to develop solutions to keep the individual patient safe. Some possible treatment solutions to wandering
behaviors may include:

- Environmental modifications: Use of signage to denote certain areas can be
  helpful in reducing wandering behaviors. This may include use of stop signs,
  "Sorry we're closed" signs, or "Do Not Enter" or "Danger" signs. Use of clear
  signage to identify a patient's room, apartment, or common areas such as the
  bathroom or dining areas also may help a patient locate areas more easily if they
  are wandering due to being lost. Use of a barrier or other camouflage to conceal
  a door also may reduce this behavior, as well as installing child-safe covers to
  doorknobs. An alarm or monitoring system may be a successful solution to
  patients living at home who are prone to leaving the house unattended.

- Use reassurance: If the patient is wandering due to "having to go to work," "pick
  up the kids from school," and so forth, refrain from correcting them. Instead try
  to validate how they feel and reassure that they can do this at another time and
  redirect them to another activity. Be sure to listen to what they are trying to tell
  you through these actions as their reasoning may lead you to better understand
  their need for the behavior in the first place.

- Increasing regular exercise: The patient may be wandering due to a need for
  movement, so increasing opportunities for regular participation in exercise may
  reduce their need to wander. If the patient follows a typical path as they move,
  provide opportunities for them to stop and engage in an activity along the
  way (e.g., a sign inviting patients to "Sit Down and Read" next to magazines/
  newspapers) or have available ways for them to stay hydrated such as a water
  station. If in a facility setting, staff should be encouraged to stop and engage
  the patient in brief conversation and possibly redirect them to another activity

if possible. Try to make the wandering purposeful by having the patient wear a pedometer to track the distance they walk each day or having parts of an activity along the patient's path that they have to gather to complete a larger task, such as gathering towels in a basket and returning to a common area to fold them.

- Increasing overall engagement in activities: If the patient is wandering because they are bored or have nothing else interesting to engage in, try to develop specific activities that cater to the patient's individual interests/hobbies. If the patient was a mechanic who also enjoyed gardening, simple activities can be created and placed in a certain area or in a separate container that cater to these interests (i.e., sorting pictures of different makes/models of cars, choosing different vegetables to be placed in a garden, etc.). These activities can be modified regularly to keep the person interested and can be developed and maintained by the patient's family if possible to increase their involvement in the patient's life and care.

- Possible goals for wandering:
  - "Patient will recall and utilize written cue indicating facility room number to reduce wandering behaviors during the initial trial of three consecutive sessions using the Spaced Retrieval technique."
  - "Patient will recall and locate personal activity box to engage in meaningful behavior and reduce wandering behaviors 80% of trials with minimal assistance."

Behavioral Challenge: Repetitive Question Asking/ Repetitive Vocalizations

Asking the same question over and over again often is cited as a top stressor for caregivers. The reason for these repetitive requests is likely due to an unmet need of either seeking information/reassurance or seeking attention. Dr. Cameron Camp (Marcell, 2006) recommends asking the patient their own question back to them to see if he/she knows the answer. If the patient does in fact know the answer to their own question, they are likely asking the question to gain attention, recognition, or reassurance. If they are unable to answer their own question, it is likely they are asking it repeatedly because they cannot recall the answer or do not recall asking the question in the first place. For example, if a patient repeatedly asks what time his daughter is coming to pick him up for his doctor appointment, the staff member can ask, "Hmm. What time do you think she is coming?" If the patient answers correctly, he is likely seeking the attention and reassurance that comes from the staff each time he asks the question. If the staff member asks, "What time do you think she is coming?" and the patient has no idea of the answer or becomes frustrated, it is likely that they do not recall the answer to the question and therefore will need a way to recall the information more independently. This may include writing down "Your daughter will pick you up at 3:00 today for your appointment" and directing the patient to read the note each time he asks a staff member the question. This will help the patient to recall the information more independently and reduce both the patient's and staff member's stress level.

Repetitive vocalizations, such as repeating over and over, "I want to go home" or "Help me, help me" can be distracting to staff, caregivers, and/or other residents/patients. Again, these vocalizations are serving some purpose for the patient, so it is important to analyze when the vocalizations are occurring as well as when they are not occurring. If the patient does not use these vocalizations when engaged in activity, then it is important to try to provide stimulation and activity as much as possible for them. If the patient seems to receive sensory stimulation from the vocalizations, providing them with headphones with music they enjoy may assist in decreasing the vocalizations. Again, asking, "Why is this behavior occurring?" will likely lead you to some possible solutions to this behavioral challenge. If the patient states that they "want to go home" repeatedly, what is it about the place they are living now that makes it not feel like home to the patient? Home often is associated less with an actual place and more with the feeling of being appreciated and needed. Providing the patient with a meaningful role within their new environment may help in making them feel more at home. Can they assist with something in the facility, like homemaking tasks, or be provided with more choice in how they spend their day? Incorporating these modifications may lead the patient to feel like they are contributing to their new home and make them feel more safe as well. Is the patient stating "help me" repeatedly due to some type of pain or because they are unaware of where they are? Checking for possible physiologic reasons and/or providing a written cue reminding them that they are safe or that family will be in to visit them soon may help to reduce the use of the phrase.

- Possible goals for repetitive question asking:
    - "Patient will recall and demonstrate use of written reminders for important information to reduce repetitive question asking behaviors and to decrease anxiety level 80% of trials during a one-week treatment period."
    - "Caregivers consistently will utilize set response to patient's repetitive question-asking behaviors to reduce patient anxiety and overall caregiver stress as evidenced by statement in daily notes in a caregiver log 80% of opportunities and demonstration of response during randomized trials during a 2-week period."

Behavioral Challenge: Decreased Intake

As persons age, their overall appetite tends to decrease. With persons with dementia, they often can forget that they need to eat or drink, which can result in weight loss and frailty. Certain medications and dental problems also can lead to a reduction in appetite (Family Caregiver Alliance, 2013). Swallowing deficits and related diet changes also can be a factor in changes in eating and appetite. It is pivotal that caregivers be aware of the patient's overall daily intake of food and liquids and address changes in them immediately. Brainstorming possible causes for decreased intake may lead to the use of the following treatment solutions:

- Diet modifications: If the patient is no longer able to eat certain foods, finding a suitable substitute may help the patient to eat more. If the patient is demonstrating difficulty using utensils to feed himself, finger foods may be substituted to allow the person to still feed themselves independently. If the patient is experiencing sensory deficits, such as a reduced sense of taste or smell, using spices or sweeteners may help them to better taste the food or cooking or baking something nearby the patient prior to a meal may help to stimulate their appetite. If the patient has a modified diet, such as a pureed diet, it may be helpful for them to sit next to others who also are on the same diet so as not to see the regular diet that they cannot safely eat. The use of commercially available food molds also can help pureed foods to take on the shape of the food they are identified with, which can help the patient find them more appetizing. Allowing the patient to choose what they wish to eat also may increase the likelihood that they will consume more and will provide them with some control over the eating experience.

- Environmental modifications: The use of proper lighting can help patients with vision issues better see the food on their plates, which can lead to increased intake. Use of contrasting plates and utensils also may help the patient to better see what they are eating (i.e., white mashed potatoes on a white plate would be difficult to see and therefore may not be eaten simply because the person was unaware that the potatoes were there). Limiting overall distractions in the dining area also can help the person with dementia to better focus on completing their meal. Presenting food in courses rather than all at once also may help someone to better focus on the eating experience and be less overwhelmed by a large amount of food served to them at one time. Offering several snacks throughout the day also may lead to an overall increase in intake rather than eating a set schedule of three meals per day. Eating with a person also can help to encourage him/her to eat more. Simply sitting next to them and encouraging them to eat can be overwhelming and demeaning. Participating in the experience with the patient makes it more enjoyable for them and for you.

- Possible goals for decreased intake:
  - "Patient will demonstrate food intake increase of 20% at two meals a day during a one-week period through caregiver use of environmental modifications to increase lighting and contrast and modifying presentation of food to patient to a maximum of two food items on plate at a time."

Summary

- The presence of behavioral symptoms in persons with dementia is common and can be challenging to the patient's caregivers.
- It is pivotal to understand that behaviors serve a purpose to the individual with dementia, and it is our job to discover what this purpose is and how we can accommodate for what the person is trying to communicate through such behaviors.

- Brainstorming with other professionals and caregivers can help in discovering the purpose behind why the person with dementia is demonstrating challenging behaviors. Trial and error at developing solutions needs to occur in order to best treat behavioral challenges.

- Skilled professionals, such as rehabilitation therapists, can be pivotal in helping to uncover why behaviors are occurring and how to treat them. Behavioral issues can be targeted during skilled therapy in the same way that other deficits may be, as long as the treating professional is explicit in how and why they are treating the behavior and additional documentation is available detailing the presence of the behavior and its overall effect on the patient's well-being and safety.

- Additional information on understanding and treating behavioral symptoms in persons with dementia can be found in the following resources:

  Bathing Without a Battle (2002), by Ann Louise Barrick, Joanne Rader, Beverly Hoeffer, and Philip Sloane, New York, NY: Springer Publishing.

  Caring for a Person with Memory Loss and Confusion: An Easy Guide for Caregivers (2002), Journeyworks Publishing, Santa Cruz, CA.

  Communicating Effectively with a Person Who Has Alzheimer's (2002), Mayo Clinic Staff, http://www.mayoclinic.com/invoke.cfm?id=AZ00004

  Steps to Enhancing Communications: Interacting with Persons with Alzheimer's Disease (1997), (Brochure) Order No. ED310Z, Alzheimer's Association, Chicago, IL.

  Steps to Understanding Challenging Behaviors: Responding to Persons with Alzheimer's Disease (1996), Alzheimer's Association, Chicago, IL.

  The Validation Breakthrough: Simple Techniques for Communicating with People with "Alzheimer's-Type Dementia," 2nd edition (2002), by Naomi Feil, Health Professions Press, Baltimore, MD.

  Understanding Difficult Behaviors: Some practical suggestions for coping with Alzheimer's Disease and Related Illnesses (2001), by A. Robinson, B. Spencer, and L. White, Eastern Michigan University, Ypsilanti, MI.

References

Alzheimer's Association. (2013a). *Treatments for behaviors*. Retrieved June 30, 2013, from http://www.alz.org/alzheimers_disease_treatments_for_behavior.asp#

Alzheimer's Association. (2013b). *Wandering and getting lost*. Retrieved June 30, 2013, from http://www.alz.org/care/alzheimers-dementia-wandering.asp

Camp, C., Cohen-Mansfield, J., & Capezuti, E. (2002). Use of nonpharmacologic interventions among nursing home residents with dementia. *Psychiatric Services, 53*(11). Retrieved June 30, 2013, from http://psychservices.psychiatryonline.org

Family Caregiver Alliance. (2013). *Caregiver's guide to understanding dementia behaviors.*

Retrieved from http://www.caregiver.org/care giver/jsp/content_node.jsp?nodeid=391

Marcell, J. (2006). *How to answer your loved one's repetitive questions.* Retrieved June 30, 2013, from http://www.healthcentral.com/alzheimers/c/43/1753/answer-loved/

Appendix 12–A

Behavior Brainstorming Worksheet (Scenario 2)

Patient: Susan F.

Challenging Behavior: Repetitive question asking to husband

Possible Reasons for Behavior (list all possible ideas): Seeking attention from husband; unable to recall answer to questions soon after receiving answer; bored throughout day (watches T.V.)

Possible Unmet Needs (circle any applicable & list why):

Physiologic _____

Love & Belonging feels ignored

Safety _____

Self-Actualization no role/input

Possible Contributory Factors (check all that apply):

_√_Environment   _√_Need for Reassurance   **Other** Unable to
_√_Routine (or lack of)   _√_Need for Social Interaction   recall answers
_√_Need for Attention   __Other Residents/Triggers

Times When Behavior Typically Occurs ("Is there a pattern?") Typically asks when husband is leaving home or engaged in something else

Times When Behavior Is Not Occurring When pt. busy with activities
Patient Aware of Behavior? __Y / _√_N

Patient's Response to Questions About Behavior: Gets frustrated; says she just "can't remember"

Previous Responses/Strategies to Reduce Behavior: Husband provides answers; gets frustrated with pt.; pt. cries in response

Possible New Strategies to Try to Reduce Behavior (list staff responsible for implementation & date to reassess): Answers to repetitive questions will be written in a notebook or on note cards near pt.'s seat in T.V. room; husband will respond to questions by directing her to the notebook/cards. Answers will be written by pt. if possible; assess activities to engage pt.; husband to provide attention/reassurance when questions not asked (SLP to provide instruction; reassess date 2 weeks from evaluation)

Rehabilitation Referral Needed: _√_Y / __N (__PT __OT _√_SLP)
Name of Staff Obtaining Referral: Jill, Home Health RN

Appendix 12–B

Behavior Brainstorming Worksheet (Scenario 3)

Patient: James B.

Challenging Behavior: Refuses to leave apt. for meals/activities

Possible Reasons for Behavior (list all possible ideas): Dislikes food; dislikes scheduled activities; dislikes table mates; depression

Possible Unmet Needs (circle any applicable & list why):

Physiologic anxiety/depression?   **Love & Belonging** feels unconnected

Safety feels someone will steal his things **Self-Actualization** no role

Possible Contributory Factors (check all that apply):

_√_Environment   __Need for Reassurance   Other
_√_Routine (or lack of)   __Need for Social Interaction
__Need for Attention   _√_Other Residents/Triggers

Times When Behavior Typically Occurs ("Is there a pattern?") Anytime staff encourages him to join for meals and/or activities

Times When Behavior Is Not Occurring Attended one current events activity & one cooking activity

Patient Aware of Behavior? _√_Y / __N

Patient's Response to Questions About Behavior: "I just don't want to be here; hate this place"

Previous Responses/Strategies to Reduce Behavior: Asking about favorite foods/favorite activities; reassurance that people are glad he's living at facility

Possible New Strategies to Try to Reduce Behavior (list staff responsible for implementation & date to reassess): Providing favorite snacks in common areas for him to eat outside of normal dining times; changing of table mates; encouraging him to observe activities/give input on activities; role of helping to implement activities rather than participate; physician referral for depression/anxiety (Activity Staff/CNAs/Nursing to implement; reassess 1 week from today)

Rehabilitation Referral Needed: __Y / _√_N (__PT __OT __SLP)
Name of Staff Obtaining Referral: N/A

Appendix 12–C

Behavior Brainstorming Worksheet (Scenario 4)

Patient: Leah V.

Challenging Behavior: Reduced intake/combativeness at meals

Possible Reasons for Behavior (list all possible ideas): Dislikes food; medication; swallowing/chewing issues; eating at other times before meals

Possible Unmet Needs (circle any applicable & list why):

Physiologic swallowing/dental; meds   **Love & Belonging**

Safety afraid may choke? pain?   **Self-Actualization**

Possible Contributory Factors (check all that apply):

_√_Environment	__Need for Reassurance	Other
__Routine (or lack of)	__Need for Social Interaction	
_√_Need for Attention	_√_Other Residents/Triggers	

Times When Behavior Typically Occurs ("Is there a pattern?") All meals except breakfast; when given desserts

Times When Behavior Is Not Occurring Breakfast
Patient Aware of Behavior? __Y / _√_N

Patient's Response to Questions About Behavior: Unresponsive or pushes food away; falls asleep at meals or tries to repeatedly get up unassisted; throws food at staff and other residents

Previous Responses/Strategies to Reduce Behavior: Providing food preferences; change of table mates

Possible New Strategies to Try to Reduce Behavior (list staff responsible for implementation & date to reassess): Dental referral; monitor food intake throughout day (snacks in room prior to meals, supplement shake given at times not near meal time; swallowing evaluation; softer foods provided if oral/dental pain(dietician consult); providing praise when eating, less attention when not (Nursing, CNAs, SLP, Dietician; reassess 2 weeks from today's date)

Rehabilitation Referral Needed: _√_Y / __N (__PT __OT _√_SLP)
Name of Staff Obtaining Referral: Laura, Director of Nursing

Appendix 12–D

Behavior Brainstorming Worksheet (Scenario 5)

Patient: Charleen C.

Challenging Behavior: Leaves adult day program unattended; wandering

Possible Reasons for Behavior (list all possible ideas): Wishes to go home; bored with activities; not sure where she needs to be

Possible Unmet Needs (circle any applicable & list why):

Physiologic   **Love & Belonging** afraid family won't pick her up

Safety feels unsafe in program **Self-Actualization** lack of engagement

Possible Contributory Factors (check all that apply):

_√_Environment   _√_Need for Reassurance   **Other**
_√_Routine (or lack of)   __Need for Social Interaction
_√_Need for Attention   _√_Other Residents/Triggers

Times When Behavior Typically Occurs ("Is there a pattern?") After being dropped off in morning; after lunch

Times When Behavior Is Not Occurring During meals; trivia activities

Patient Aware of Behavior? _√_Y / __N

Patient's Response to Questions About Behavior: Wants to go home; afraid family won't be able to find her; unable to answer what time she is picked up

Previous Responses/Strategies to Reduce Behavior: Seated away from main doors; redirection into activities; change of door code number

Possible New Strategies to Try to Reduce Behavior (list staff responsible for implementation & date to reassess): Visual cue on walker of daughter's picture with time she is being picked up; speech therapy for recall of visual cue & staff follow-through; positive reinforcement when engaged in activity; individualized trivia activities when dropped off and after lunch; staff reassurance

Rehabilitation Referral Needed: _√_Y / __N (__PT __OT _√_SLP)
Name of Staff Obtaining Referral: Susan, Director of Activities

Appendix 12–E

Behavior Brainstorming Worksheet (Scenario 6)

Patient: Craig M.

Challenging Behavior: Combative during bathing

Possible Reasons for Behavior (list all possible ideas): Afraid of bathing process; unaware of need to bathe/timing of baths; fear of being hurt

Possible Unmet Needs (circle any applicable & list why):

Physiologic   **Love & Belonging** unable to recognize staff

Safety feels unsafe   **Self-Actualization**

Possible Contributory Factors (check all that apply):

_√_Environment   __Need for Reassurance   **Other**
__Routine (or lack of)   __Need for Social Interaction
__Need for Attention   _√_Other Residents/Triggers

Times When Behavior Typically Occurs ("Is there a pattern?") Anytime bathing is initiated; becomes agitated with staff member Brian

Times When Behavior Is Not Occurring When Jessica, R.N. assists
Patient Aware of Behavior? _√_Y / __N

Patient's Response to Questions About Behavior: "Don't need a bath."; "Leave me alone"; "No man is giving me a bath"

Previous Responses/Strategies to Reduce Behavior: Environmental changes to bathroom; shower vs. bath; time of day of bath, after breakfast bath successful at times

Possible New Strategies to Try to Reduce Behavior (list staff responsible for implementation & date to reassess): Provide large-print name tags for staff assisting to orient pt.; prepare pt. for bathing experience (towels on bed after breakfast; state reason towels are present); speak with Jessica about her strategies that reassure pt.(Nursing; CNAs; Jessica; housekeeping; reassess 2 weeks from today)

Rehabilitation Referral Needed: __Y / _√_N (__PT __OT __SLP)
Name of Staff Obtaining Referral: N/A

Appendix 12–F

Behavior Brainstorming Worksheet (Scenario 7)

Patient: Bill S.

Challenging Behavior: Tries to get out of bed/chair unattended frequently in room

Possible Reasons for Behavior (list all possible ideas): Forgets need for assistance; urgency of need (get to bathroom); forgets hip precautions/safety needs; bored (needs attention/interaction)

Possible Unmet Needs (circle any applicable & list why):

Physiologic frequent need to use bathroom **Love & Belonging**

Safety feels staff won't assist in time **Self-Actualization** bored

Possible Contributory Factors (check all that apply):

_√_Environment   __Need for Reassurance   Other
__Routine (or lack of)   _√_Need for Social Interaction
_√_Need for Attention   __Other Residents/Triggers

Times When Behavior Typically Occurs ("Is there a pattern?") Between lunch and dinner (after PT); middle of night

Times When Behavior Is Not Occurring When not in room alone; visitors
Patient Aware of Behavior? _√_Y / __N

Patient's Response to Questions About Behavior: "I forgot I needed help"; "I couldn't find call button"; "I had to use restroom"; "I don't know why I hit the button for you"

Previous Responses/Strategies to Reduce Behavior: Set bathroom/toileting schedule; instruction on hip precautions; relocating call button

Possible New Strategies to Try to Reduce Behavior (list staff responsible for implementation & date to reassess): Urology consult; assess meds; set schedule to check on pt. at regular intervals day/night for social interaction/bathroom assist (if needed); SLP referral to teach call button use/recall of hip precautions; PT/OT to evaluate safety needs/adaptive equipment; provide individual activities in room to engage pt. (Nursing, CNAs, PT, OT, SLP, housekeeping, dietary, activities staff)

Rehabilitation Referral Needed: _√_Y / __N (_√_PT _√_OT _√_SLP)
Name of Staff Obtaining Referral: Kelsey, Director of Nursing

138

13

Drugs and Supplements

Pharmacological Intervention

As of the printing of this book, there is no cure for nonreversible dementia (i.e., Alzheimer's disease). There is no "quick fix" and no magic pill to stop the disease or reverse the damage to the brain cells caused by deterioration. There are some medications available that work to control the symptoms but will not reverse the disease process. In addition, there have been numerous claims that certain dietary supplements or vitamin regimes will reverse the symptoms of dementia. While there may be some validity to these claims, it is not our job as SLPs to prescribe any treatment for dementia or recommend medications or supplements. It is helpful to know about the different drug options available so that we can identify side effects that affect our treatment and a patient's progress. The following is information about drug regimens available today. This chapter gives a brief overview of some of the medications and alternative treatments used for dementia.

Types of Drugs

There are two types of drugs approved by the United States Food and Drug Administration for dementia: cholinesterase inhibitors and memantine. These drugs do not work for all individuals. Some may demonstrate improvement in function and a reduction in symptoms, while others will continue to deteriorate.

The beneficial effects of these drugs may not appear for several weeks or even months.

Cholinesterase Inhibitors

Alzheimer research has shown that there is a decrease in the level of acetylcholine, a chemical messenger that assists with memory, thought, and judgment in the brain. Cholinesterase inhibitors were developed to improve the effectiveness of acetylcholine in the brain by slowing the breakdown of this chemical and increasing levels improving communication between nerve cells. The most common drugs in the class prescribed are Donepezil (Aricept), Galantamine (Reminyl), Rivastigmine (Exelon), and Tacrine (Cognex). In cases where these drugs have been effective, patients and caregivers reported a slowing in symptoms such as memory loss, reduced anxiety, improved mood, and restored confidence levels (Merck & Company, 1997).

Common side effects of these drugs include nausea, vomiting, diarrhea, and lack of muscle coordination, which can affect balance. Infrequent side effects include rash, indigestion, headache, muscle aches, loss of appetite, stomach pain, nervousness, chills, dizziness, drowsiness, dry or itching eyes, increased sweating, joint pain, runny nose, sore throat, swelling of feet or legs, insomnia, weight loss, unusual tiredness or weakness, and flushing of the face (Griffith, 2004). This is not a complete list of side effects and others may occur.

Once a patient stops taking a drug, their condition will deteriorate during a period of four to six weeks until they are at the same point as an individual who has not taken the drug. Once administration of this medication stops, it is not possible to regain prior cognitive function from when the medication was taken in the past. This is an important point that most caregivers are unaware of when they are making a decision to stop medications.

Memantine

Memantine is in a class of medications called NMDA receptor antagonists. It works by decreasing abnormal activity in the brain by binding to NMDA receptors on brain cells and blocking the activity of the neurotransmitter glutamate. At normal levels, glutamate aids in memory and learning, but if levels are too high, glutamate appears to overstimulate and thus kill the nerve cells (Merck & Company, 1997).

Common side effects of memantine include nausea, vomiting, diarrhea, constipation, loss of appetite, dizziness, weight loss, swelling of hands or feet, rapid heart rate, skin rash, joint pain, redness or swelling of or around the eyes, anxiety, aggression, easy bruising or bleeding, unusual weakness, and urinating more than usual. This is not a complete list of side effects and others may occur (Merck & Company, 1997).

Just as with the cholinesterase inhibitors, it may take a few weeks of dosing to see effects of this drug. In addition, if the drug is stopped, cognitive and/or behavioral deterioration may occur and may not be recouped if the drug is reinstated at a later time.

Medications for Behavioral Symptoms

The diagnosis of dementia rarely is suffered in isolation of any other diagnosis. It usually is accompanied by a number of other comorbidities, many of which are psychiatric. Some examples may include anxiety, depression, delirium, and so forth. Some of these behavioral comorbidities may be a manifestation of the medication that is prescribed for the dementia and additional medication then is prescribed on top of the dementia medication to treat the side effects. You can see how complicated pharmacological intervention can be with someone who has dementia. We will not attempt to go into detail about the interventions for all of the symptoms associated with dementia but want clinicians to understand the relationship between pharmacological intervention and behaviors that may impede progress in therapy.

Drugs prescribed to treat anxiety and/or depression and other behaviors sometimes may cause reactions of drowsiness and excessive fatigue (Griffith, 2004). These reactions in turn may affect a patient's ability to attend to tasks in therapy, function well during tasks of daily living, and may affect balance and coordination causing an increase in falls. These drugs also may affect mood with increased irritability, aggressiveness, and appetite reduction.

If you see behaviors that may be negatively affecting progress, functioning of activities of daily living, or are having a negative impact on the communication and interaction with family or caregivers, it is important to communicate these behaviors with the patient's physician. The physician ultimately will be responsible for determining if the behavior is associated as a medication side effect or an effect of a combination of drugs. The physician may consult with you or the family member to determine if a change in drug regimen is indicated. Changing the drug regimen can be taxing on the patient as there often are side effects that can occur with a subtle change in dosing. Therefore, frequent medication changes and alterations in the dosing often is discouraged.

Non-Pharmocological Intervention

It is helpful to know about some of the alternative therapies that can be considered for the treatment of dementia. Many of the dietary supplements and herbal remedies are not monitored by the federal Food and Drug Administration and are not recommended by professional medical organizations. Much of the information that family members receive about alternative treatments is gleaned from the internet and offer little or no research or investigative data to back the claims for effective treatment of dementia. Whether a treatment is valid or not, it is not the SLP's responsibility to back or reject a claim, and the clinician needs to be very cautious in offering advice or guidance regarding pursuit of any intervention. The following is a list of dietary supplements provided by the Alzheimer's Association.

Caprylic Acid and Coconut Oil

Caprylic acid is a triglyceride that is the active ingredient in Axona, a drug marketed as a "medical food." It is produced in processing coconut and palm oil (Alzheimer's Association, 2013). The use of caprylic acid or coconut oil has not been proven to be effective in the treatment of Alzheimer's; however, there are numerous articles and reports found on the Internet reporting on improved cognition following a regimen of coconut oil.

Coenzyme Q10

Coenzyme Q10, or ubiquinone, is an antioxidant that naturally occurs in the body and is needed for normal cell reactions (Alzheimer's Association, 2013). This compound has not been studied for its effectiveness in treating Alzheimer's. Idebenone is a synthetic version of this compound and once was tested for Alzheimer's disease but showed little or no effectiveness. The Alzheimer's Association stresses that little is known about safe dosages of coenzyme Q10 and further, as with many other supplements, there could be harmful effects if too much is taken (Alzheimer's Association, 2013).

Ginkgo Biloba

The herb, ginkgo biloba, has been used medicinally for thousands of years and is thought to have antioxidant and anti-inflammatory properties. According to the Mayo Clinic, there is research in the efficacy of using this herb to treat Alzheimer's disease and multi-infarct dementia (MID). The Mayo Clinic further reports "although not definitive, there is promising early evidence favoring the use of Ginkgo for memory enhancement in health subjects" (Mayo Clinic, 2012). According to the Alzheimer's Association, researchers have found no difference between groups that have taken ginkgo and those given a placebo (Alzheimer's Association, 2013).

Huperzine A

Huperzine A is a dietary supplement extracted from Chinese club moss that reacts similarly to cholinesterase inhibitors. There are some studies that suggest that its use may protect memory and retard cognitive decline in Alzheimer's patients. There is no research on long-term effects and the Alzheimer's Association lists a number of medications that should be avoided if taking Huperzine A (Mayo Clinic, 2012).

Omega 3 Fatty Acids

Omega 3s are a type of polyunsaturated fat that have been linked to a reduction of heart disease and stroke. There also has been a link to a possible reduction in cognitive decline or dementia. The Alzheimer's Association summarizes a couple of promising studies on the effects of high doses of Omega 3s on dementia; however, it also states that much more research is needed to support this supplement as a viable treatment (Alzheimer's Association, 2013).

Be Cautiously Supportive

There are dozens of other dietary supplements found on various websites claiming successful treatment of dementia symptoms. Our patients and their loved ones often will turn to the Internet for information and possible "cures" for the disease. We cannot interfere with their Internet searches, and the best approach is to support the family in doing thorough investigation into the treatment and obtaining second and third opinions. Most importantly, it is imperative to encourage medical supervision while attempting any intervention that may affect the patient's physical or behavioral status.

Clinical Trials

There have been some fascinating research and discovery about Alzheimer's disease and other dementias during the past couple of decades, and there will continue to be a need for research well into the future. Clinical trials are a way for patients with dementia and/or caregivers and family members to take part in this research. By signing up for a clinical trial, patients may have the opportunity to receive cutting-edge treatment and/or medications without cost. Of course, there can be a number of risks involved in participating in clinical trials, which is for the patient and/or family member to decide if the risk is worth the benefits. If you think your patient may be interested in participating, the Alzheimer's Association has information on how to become a participant in a clinical trial (Alzheimer's Association, 2013).

References

Alzheimer's Association. (2013). *Alternative treatments*. Retrieved March 2, 2013, from http://www.alz.org

Griffith, H. W. (2004). *Complete guide to prescription and nonprescription drugs*. New York, NY: Berkley.

Mayo Clinic. (2012). *Mayo Clinic drugs and supplements*. Retrieved March 2, 2013, from http://www.mayoclinic.com

Merck & Company. (1997). *The Merck Manual of Medical Information*. New York, NY: Simon and Schuster.

14

The Holistic Approach

Working with the dementia population is an undertaking that cannot be done in isolation. No matter what setting you are working in, it is important to work within the context of a team in order to provide the patients and their families with the most effective treatment and care. The best approach to the care of individuals affected by dementia includes support from multiple sources. These may be integrated, parallel, or a combination of both (Grand, Caspar, & MacDonald, 2011). This chapter discusses the specific roles of the members of a dementia care team, and how the speech-language pathologist (SLP) or other rehabilitation professional can implement co-treatment ideas to best serve the needs of the patient.

Dementia Care Team Members

There are a number of professionals who can be members of a patient's care team. Communication and collaboration among all of these professionals is paramount to good patient care. Here we will share the most common members of a dementia care team and highlight their roles and overall scope of practice. Detailed descriptions of each discipline's scope of practice may be found on each governing body's Web site, such as the American Physical Therapy Association and the American Speech-Language-Hearing Association. This list is not exhaustive; as with each patient, specific professionals may be needed based on the patient's additional diagnoses and needs.

- Physicians: As we have discussed, a patient's physician is the main point of contact for all other professionals working with an individual with dementia. A patient's team of physicians may include the primary care physician, along with additional specialists such as a neurologist, geriatrician, psychiatrist, and other specialists the patient may see for additional diagnoses, such as a cardiologist, oncologist, or orthopedist. In a facility setting, the patient's care may be overseen by a medical director for the facility or the patient may choose to have their care monitored by an outside physician. In any case, it is important for the professional working with the dementia patient to be aware of who the primary physicians are in a patient's care in order to request and receive orders for treatment and changes in care.

- Registered nurse (RN)/licensed practical nurse (LPN): Most patients in a facility setting will have nursing staff who are charged with administering and monitoring the patient's overall Plan of Care. The nursing staff at skilled facilities typically administer medications and other treatments, such as wound care. In home settings, an RN or LPN working for a home healthcare agency may be the case manager, overseeing the patient's overall care and the implementation of the patient's Plan of Care. In settings such as assisted living facilities, a RN may act as a director of nursing, overseeing all patient care, while the LPNs perform the daily care routines with the patient such as administering medications. Nurses from a home care agency may be ordered by the physician to perform more skilled procedures, such as wound care and catheter changes and maintenance.

- Social worker: A licensed social worker performs many duties related to the care of the individual with dementia. This discipline may work in the hospital setting, a skilled nursing facility, an assisted living facility, or through a home healthcare agency. The social worker in a hospital setting typically assists patients and their families with planning for their discharge either to a facility or to the home setting. They provide options to the patient and their families as to the best fit for the level of care the patient needs and assists with the needed referrals for the patient for when they leave the hospital setting as part of discharge planning. Social workers are advocates for the patients and can provide resources to patients and families regarding support groups, counseling, community outreach programs, available programs, such as Meals on Wheels, and information on assistance programs. Many times in facility settings, the social workers are the main point of contact for the families in understanding and participating in their loved one's care. They are members of the interdisciplinary team serving the patient.

- Registered dietician (RD): A licensed dietician oversees the nutritional health of the patient. The dietician will review the patient's overall intake of both food and liquids and make recommendations to the physician if the patient is at risk for malnutrition or dehydration. The dietician works closely with the SLP if a patient is experiencing swallowing difficulties and requires a change in diet consistency in order to safely eat or drink.

- Physical therapist (PT): According to the Mayo Clinic, physical therapists: "work with patients who have impairments, limitations, disabilities, or changes in physical function and health status resulting from injury, disease, or other causes. Their role includes examination, evaluation, diagnosis, prognosis, and interventions toward achieving the highest functional outcomes for each patient/

client" (Mayo Clinic, 2013). PTs develop treatment plans related to the patient's specific physical needs, such as after-care for a hip or knee replacement or balance issues. Physical therapy assistants (PTAs) may be overseen by a PT to implement the recommended Plan of Care. PTs may be found in any setting that cares for an individual with dementia.

- Occupational therapist (OT): According to the American Occupational Therapy Association (AOTA), OTs working with the dementia population "evaluate persons with dementia to determine their strengths, impairments, and performance areas needing intervention" (Schaber & Lieberman, 2010). These performance areas needing intervention may be fine motor skills, rehabilitation of the upper extremities, transferring skills (such as transferring from sit to stand or stand to sit), accommodations for visual deficits, and recommendation and implementation of modifications to the patient's environment or use of adaptive equipment to maintain safety and function (AOTA, 2013). Like PTs, OTs can be found in any setting that treats and cares for persons with dementia and can have assistants or COTAs (certified occupational therapy assistants) to implement treatment.

- Speech-language pathologist (SLP): According to the American Speech-Language-Hearing Association (ASHA), SLPs play a primary role in the screening, assessment, diagnosis, treatment, and research of cognitive-communication disorders, including those associated with dementia. This may include treatment of cognitive deficits, swallowing difficulties, and overall reduced communication skills. ASHA further details that the primary roles of the SLP working with the dementia population include identification, assessment, intervention, counseling, collaboration, case management, education, advocacy, and research (ASHA, 2005).

- Audiologist: According to the American-Speech-Language-Hearing Association, the practice of audiology "includes both the prevention of and assessment of auditory, vestibular, and related impairments as well as the habilitation/ rehabilitation and maintenance of persons with these impairments" (ASHA, 2004). With the dementia population, the audiologist primarily would assess, treat, and monitor any hearing or vestibular impairments and oversee the use and maintenance of the patient's hearing aids.

- Certified nursing assistant (CNA): CNAs are trained to safely bathe, groom, dress, and assist patients with their ADLs (activities of daily living). They also are trained to safely assist with ambulation, transfers, and bed mobility. In addition, the CNAs may provide active and passive range of motion (ROM) exercises and are educated to provide patients with basic massage such as back rubs and skin care to prevent breakdown. The CNA also learns about nutrition and basic anatomy and physiology (Quan, 2012). CNAs often are the discipline that regularly sees the patient throughout the day, are key in implementing the patient's Plan of Care, and are the "eyes and ears" for the rest of the interdisciplinary team and the family as to how the patient is functioning.

- Activity directors/recreational therapist: Geriatric activities directors facilitate recreational and therapeutic activities in nursing homes, senior centers, and residential facilities. Geriatric activities directors plan and facilitate games and sports, create arts and crafts projects, and organize entertainment events like concerts and plays. They also design and create individualized activities for patients in order to keep them actively engaged throughout the day. Like the CNAs, these professionals also can be the "eyes and ears" for the rest of the care team as to how the patient is functioning and participating in everyday life.

Collaboration and Co-Treatment

Collaboration among all professionals working with the patient with dementia is key to successful care. Formal collaboration meetings may occur regularly in some settings, while informal discussions about a patient's care typically are ongoing. However these communications occur, it is important that they do, as each discipline plays a specific role in working with the patient and their family. It can be difficult at times to coordinate a patient's care as effectively as we would like due to productivity requirements, scheduling differences, and so forth, but it is pivotal that a system be put into place to allow each member of the care team to communicate with one another and to document this communication regularly to insure that all of the needs of the patient are being met and that follow-through on recommendations is completed. At the very least, we recommend that each professional documents on their treatment notes or in the patient's chart, if applicable, any discussions that occur among the team members and expected outcomes of these discussions as these are key elements that state and corporate auditors as well as Medicare reviewers look for when reviewing a patient's overall care. As the saying goes, "if it wasn't documented, it didn't happen," so make sure that your documentation reflects any and all collaboration and communication you do.

Co-treatment can be defined as "more than one professional providing treatment during the same session" (White, 2009). Although collaboration among professionals is recommended, it is important to note that co-treatment, particularly related to rehabilitation services, like physical, occupational, and speech therapy, must be monitored closely and implemented with an awareness of how the treatments will be documented and submitted for billing and reimbursement. For example, for a patient with dementia who also has dysphagia (swallowing deficits) and motor planning and fine motor deficits, the patient would benefit from the services of both a speech-language pathologist (SLP) and an occupational therapist (OT). It may serve the patient best to have both professionals work with the patient at the same time during a meal so that the SLP can focus on the patient's swallowing skills and diet tolerance, while the OT addresses the fine motor needs for self-feeding. According to ASHA, co-treatment billing should be viewed by the patient's time receiving the service not by the provider's time giving the service (White, 2009). This rule also has been adopted by Medicare. In other words, if the patient is seen for a one-hour session by both the OT and the SLP, the OT and SLP should calculate their billing time by how long the patient receives direct service from them individually, perhaps 30 minutes each, and not each bill for one hour of service to the patient. It also is important that services do not overlap in any way; meaning that if the OT is billing for instruction and treatment for transfers, the PT cannot bill for that service as well. We mention this here as we want to encourage all disciplines on the dementia care team to work collaboratively and in conjunction with another as often as possible, while keeping in mind the importance of the ethical considerations for billing for services.

Collaboration also can be accomplished by each discipline noting deficits they see in a patient that may be best served by another discipline. For example, a home care nurse may be working with a patient on understanding their medications but due to the patient's dementia has noticed that the patient is not retaining the education being provided during their visits. The nurse then may ask for a referral from the physician for speech therapy to help the patient recall the information being taught by the nurse and for recommendations on how to modify the educational materials so that the patient may better benefit from them. The nurse also may ask for occupational therapy to see the patient to work on adapting the environment and the patient's pillbox so that the patient can access his medications more easily. In this example, all three disciplines would be seeing a patient for medication adherence, but all would be seeing the patient specifically related to their own scope of practice. Clear documentation of what each discipline does with the patient in the sessions along with clear goals highlighting these areas allow for the patient to benefit from the expertise of all three disciplines while not billing for the same focus of service.

Collaborative Treatment Guide

Here we list some functional ways the different members of the dementia care team can work together to serve the needs of the patient. These ideas not only allow for the better and more connected care for the patient but also for the team members to be creative and have fun working together, as well.

- Activity creation (Team members: Recreational therapist, OT, SLP, patient families): The recreational therapist may wish to develop specific individualized activities for some of the residents of the facility but may not have the time or resources to do so. The recreational therapist could ask the families of the patients to bring in magazines and catalogs, which then are passed along to the occupational therapist. The OT then would have patients who are working on fine motor skills cut out pictures from the magazines/catalogs and glue the pictures to index cards as part of their OT sessions. These cards then are given to the SLP who would have her patients sort the pictures into categories, work on descriptions of the pictures, and so forth to work on speech and language skills during their speech sessions. The cards then are given to the recreational therapist to use with the residents in individual activities to have the patients sort the cards based on their own interests.

- External/visual cues (Team members: PT, OT, SLP, CNAs): The physical therapist may notice during treatment that a patient with dementia is regularly using his walker incorrectly, making it difficult for him to make progress in physical therapy. The PT may ask the OT to develop a simple visual cue for the patient's walker to remind him of how to use the walker to accommodate for his visual deficits. The SLP may work with the patient in treatment to recall that the visual cue is on the walker and what the cue means using a technique like Spaced Retrieval (see Chapter 9). The PT then would monitor if the patient is effectively using the walker safely as a result of the presence of the visual cue and the speech therapy to help the patient recall its presence on the walker. The CNAs then would monitor and document if the patient is safely using the walker outside of his therapy sessions.

- Dining (Team members: SLP, OT, PT, CNA, Nurse, Dietician): The facility nurse and CNAs begin to notice several residents who are eating and drinking less during meals. Upon requesting referrals from the residents' physicians for evaluations from speech and occupational therapies, the patients are deemed to have varying reasons for their decreased intake, including swallowing difficulties and fine motor, visual, and perceptual deficits. It is discovered that several of the patients also are being seen by physical therapy for difficulty with ambulation. The SLP, OT, and dietician collaborate on the patient's nutritional needs and establish a "Walk to Dine" program with PT to address ambulation to and from meals. All of the involved disciplines work within their individual scopes of practice to treat the patients for their individual needs within the functional activity of dining.

- Home organization (Team members: OT, SLP, CNA, family): A patient with dementia is being seen by a home health agency for compensatory memory strategies and home safety needs. The OT and SLP work with the patient and his family to establish a better sense of order for the materials the patient uses each day, including personal hygiene items, clothing, and leisure activity items, to increase safety and reduce fall risk. The OT teaches the patient to use adaptive equipment to better access the materials, while the SLP works with the patient to sort the items into categories, label them with simple, easy-to-follow instructions, problem solve the best placement of the materials in the home, and recall their locations. The CNA and family work under the direction and instructions of the OT and SLP to encourage the patient to use his adaptive equipment and recall where materials are and how to use them independently rather than relying on the family to locate and help him use the materials.

- Effective activities (Team members: SLP and recreational therapist): The SLP may collaborate with the recreational therapist on how to improve implementation of activities within the facility setting to accommodate the varying needs of the patients with dementia. This may include how to easily and simply state directions, how to use visual cueing to accommodate for memory deficits, and how to create and implement activities that capitalize on the patient's strengths and abilities. The SLP may be treating patients in skilled therapy sessions but can see how well the patients participate in the group activities as part of generalization and carryover of skills. Likewise, the recreational therapist can recommend activity ideas to the SLP to use during individual treatment that the patients enjoy, which can incorporate the patients' speech therapy goals to make the treatment more fun and meaningful for the patients.

Summary

- Care of the patient with dementia should be a team approach. All disciplines involved in the ongoing care of the patient should communicate and collaborate regularly with one another in order to best serve the needs of the patient and their families.

- There are many members to a good dementia care team. This may include physicians, nurses, rehabilitation therapists, dieticians, social workers, and certified nursing assistants. All are valuable members of the team and have different scopes of practice to utilize in the care of the patient.

- Co-treatment and collaboration also are elements of good dementia care. Professionals should look at patient deficits from a holistic perspective, analyzing each issue and finding ways that each discipline can assist in managing the difficulties the patient may face throughout the course of dementia. This can allow for the care to be creative and fun while providing the most benefit to the patient.

References

American Occupational Therapy Association (AOTA). (2013). *Dementia and the role of occupational therapy.* Retrieved June 30, 2013, from http://www.aota.org/Consumers/Professionals/WhatIsOT/PA/Facts/Dementia.aspx

American Speech-Language-Hearing Association (ASHA). (2004). *Scope of practice in audiology.* Retrieved June 30, 2013, from http://www.asha.org/policy

American Speech-Language-Hearing Association (ASHA). (2005). *The roles of speech-language pathologists working with individuals with dementia-based communication disorders: Position statement* [Position statement]. Retrieved June 30, 2013, from http://www.asha.org/policy

Grand, J., Caspar, S., & MacDonald, S. (2011). Clinical features and multidisciplinary approaches to dementia care. *Journal of Multidisciplinary Healthcare, 4,* 125–147.

Mayo Clinic. (2013). *Physical therapy.* Retrieved June 30, 2013, from http://www.mayo.edu/mshs/careers/physical-therapy

Quan, K. (2012). *Understanding the critical role certified nursing assistants play in patient care.* Retrieved June 30, 2013, from http://www .nursetogether.com/understanding-the-criti cal-role-certified-nursing-assistants-play-in-patient-care

Schaber, P., & Lieberman, D. (2010). *Occupational therapy practice guidelines for adults with Alzheimer's disease and related disorders.* Bethesda, MD: AOTA Press.

White, S. C. (2009). Bottom line: Billing for co-treatment. *The ASHA Leader.*

15

Special Considerations for the Home Health Therapist

Home. To most people, this is the place where we feel the most comfortable. The place where you feel safe, the place where all of the things and people you love are found. Home also is the setting where many patients with dementia now are being treated. According to the National Association for Home Care & Hospice (2010), approximately 12 million individuals and their families currently receive care in their homes from more than 33,000 providers, including the services of a speech-language pathologist (SLP). With the onset of shortened hospital stays and the patients' strong desires to remain in their homes for as long as possible, many older adults and their families are turning to home care providers to receive rehabilitative services. Because this care setting is becoming increasingly more popular for patients and their families, we feel it is important to provide treating professionals with a brief overview of the home care setting and the special considerations for practicing in this setting. This chapter highlights those considerations to prepare professionals who may choose to work in home health care and to provide support to those who currently are working in it.

What Is Home Health Care?

Home health care is a service delivery option for patients who are recovering from an illness, undergoing treatment for an illness, or are disabled, chronically ill, or terminally ill. Patients seen in home care also must meet the definition for being homebound. According to Medicare (2013), the definition of homebound includes the following: due to the patient's condition, leaving home is not recommended, the patient's condition keeps him/her from leaving home without help (such as using a wheelchair or walker, needing special transportation, or getting help from another person), and leaving home takes a considerable and taxing effort. A person may leave home for short durations of time for medical treatment or to attend religious services, but these must be limited in frequency. A patient's physician may recommend the services of a home healthcare agency for patients who fit this definition, even if the patient only meets the criteria for being home-bound for a limited amount of time, such as after a hip replacement. Home care agencies provide the services of skilled nursing, rehabilitation services, home health aides, medical social workers, and a number of other services.

There are a number of reasons why a patient may need or would benefit from home health care. These include postsurgical care (such as following a hip or knee replacement); post-acute rehabilitation (such as after a stroke); treatment of ongoing, progressive illness (Parkinson's disease, Alzheimer's disease, or cancer); or following injury (hip or fractured hip). The overall adult population seen in home care typically is more medically acute and fragile, is more culturally diverse, and can have a wide range of disorders (Malone & Loehr, 2013).

The three main options for reimbursement for home health care include Medicare, private insurance, and private payment. Medicare is the most common provider of coverage to home health care. Patients who are covered under Part A Medicare benefits and qualify as needing a skilled service can receive home health care covered at 100% reimbursement without a co-pay. Medicare payment to the home health agency is determined according to the level and complexity of services needed to care for the patient. The skill level is determined at the time of the initial evaluation (completed by a SLP, physical therapist, or registered nurse) and is submitted to Medicare for reimbursement. This system is called the prospective payment system (PPS), familiar to many who have experience working in the skilled nursing facilities. It is named prospective payment because it occurs before services to the patient are rendered. If services are terminated early, or not delivered according to the plan submitted by the home health agency, the agency must reimburse Medicare a portion of the payment (Malone & Loehr, 2013).

Another form of reimbursement for home health services is private insurance. This coverage can vary greatly from one company to the next. In general, after the insurance company authorizes services, they reimburse a percentage of the total bill, with the patient responsible for the remainder of the costs. Some insurance companies will reimburse similar to that of Medicare and will cover 100% of the services (Malone & Loehr, 2013). Very few patients choose to pay for home care services out of pocket as it can be very costly.

The OASIS and Reassessment Requirements

The Outcome and Assessment Information Set (OASIS) is the evaluation tool used by the home health industry to assess the needs of its patients in order to develop an appropriate Plan of Care and determine reimbursement. The home health industry uses the tool to assess or make alterations to services during the course of care. Care providers complete different OASIS forms at different phases of care, including the admission, resumption of care, and at a point of discharge, or if the patient is transferred to acute care. The OASIS forms are composed of numerous multiple choice and fill-in-the-blank questions that pertain to area such as diagnoses, pain assessment, change in condition, medication assessment (including drug interactions), activities of daily living function including communication, mobility, feeding, toileting, grooming, and hygiene, multisystem status (respiratory, skin integrity, cardiovascular, urinary status, and nutrition), cognition and behavior, psychosocial status, and community resource involvement (Malone & Loehr, 2013).

At this time, only skilled nurses, PTs, and SLPs may complete the OASIS assessments. It requires specific training to complete and can be daunting to the unfamiliar professional. It requires the assessing professionals to be able to look at a patient's complete set of needs and to make referrals for additional disciplines and services, if needed.

Medicare now requires that regular therapy reassessments be conducted throughout the patient's service period. This means that the patient must be reassessed at specific visits (by the 13th and 19th visits) by the skilled professional(s) (PT, OT, SLP), and that the visits are cumulative, meaning that all of the therapy visits are combined to reach the specified visits. As of January 2013, the therapy reassessment guidelines read "reassessment visits are completed during the 11th, 12th, or 13th Medicare-covered therapy visit for the required 13th visit reassessment and the 17th, 18th, or 19th visit for the required 19th visit reassessment" (CMS, 2013). It is very important for these reassessments to occur or the entire episode of care may not be covered by Medicare.

Plan of Care and Goal Considerations

A Plan of Care (POC) is comprised of short-term and long-term goals. The home health SLP must submit this plan and a plan for treatment frequency to the physician for approval. Long-term and short-term goals are included in the assessment and reassessment documentation. Documentation of functional progress must be evident and clearly stated on daily notes and 60-day reassessments in order for treatment to continue. Long-term goals generally are set at 60-day intervals because reimbursement for care covers a 60-day period. Once this period is complete, the team completes a re-certification OASIS and treatment reassessments and updates or establishes short-term and long-term goals (Malone & Loehr, 2013).

The POC also entails determining the number of treatment visits and the frequency that those visits should be made in order for the patient to benefit and make progress in meeting goals. This is called frequency and duration of visits. The frequency refers to how many times a week the patient will receive treatment services, and the duration refers to how many weeks they will be receiving treatment. For example, a patient may be evaluated by an SLP and it is determined that they will need eight visits of therapy. The SLP may write the frequency and duration for this treatment to be twice a week for four weeks, twice a week for three weeks and once a week for two weeks, or three times a week for two weeks and once a week for two weeks, and so forth. The frequency and duration are determined based on a number of areas, which first and foremost include the patient's needs, but they also can include the frequency and intensity of services from other disciplines, family and patient requests, and scheduling considerations.

The home health SLP prioritizes goal areas based on the patient's need and may treat several related issues simultaneously. For example, a patient may be referred for a swallowing problem but also may have a compounding cognitive-linguistic deficit that impacts following instructions or using compensatory strategies. Many times, home care patients are authorized by their insurance to receive a limited number of sessions, so the SLP must be realistic in setting goals and efficient in implementing treatment.

Keeping the patient safe and functioning as independently as possible are priority goal areas for patients being treated in their homes. Regularly tying goals to the patient's overall safety can help the treatment plan remain as functional as possible. Home exercise programs, such as those prescribed by physical and occupational therapists, need to be completed regularly by the patient in order for progress to be made. Similarly, SLPs may recommend swallowing home exercise programs be completed regularly in order to maintain or improve swallow function. Goals related to home exercise programs must be detailed and allow for both the patient and their caregivers (if applicable) to show return demonstration of the exercises to the therapist. This will help insure that the patient and caregivers know what is expected of them in order for functional change to occur.

Challenges of the Home Care Environment

Treating a patient in their home can be very meaningful and functional for the patient. Professionals treating a patient in the home setting are afforded the opportunity to see the patient in the environment in which they function each and every day. Patients typically are more comfortable in their own homes and can be very motivated to participate in treatment. Patients with dementia are no exception. In fact, many of these patients perform better in treatment in their homes because it is such a familiar environment to them and encompasses so many familiar routines for them. However, treating the patient with dementia in their own home does present with some challenges. If the patient is living alone without regular family or outside assistance, the home care therapist may be the only person seeing and interacting with the patient on a regular basis. This means that the home care therapist must assess the patient's overall living situation and safety on a regular basis and notify others (family, physician, etc.) if the patient no longer is safely living in their home. This also means that the home care therapist must be aware of local agencies to connect the patient and/or their family with if additional assistance is needed, such as a companion service, house cleaning, or food delivery. If the patient is living with family, but it is suspected that the patient is not being well taken care of or abused in anyway (physically, emotionally, financially), the proper authorities such as Adult Protective Services must be notified. This can be a large burden and undertaking for the home care professional, but it is a necessary part of service delivery in this setting.

Noncompliance and Family Considerations

Although motivation for treatment can be high in home care, noncompliance with treatment recommendations also may occur. Because these patients often are medically fragile, they may fatigue easily. Home care patients often are recovering from a recent stay in a hospital or skilled nursing facility and, therefore, may become overwhelmed by the number of disciplines treating them, leading to the refusal of treatment visits or failure to follow-through with recommended treatment activities and strategies. Thobaben (2007) feels certain characteristics are typical of patients who are noncompliant with treatment. These include an overall failure to progress in treatment areas (evidenced by performance on objective tests or behavior that is indicative of failure to adhere to the overall treatment plan), an exacerbation of symptoms, and development of complications. Thobaben (2007) also examined possible reasons for noncompliance in home care patients, such as discomfort from treatment; medication side effects; worries regarding the expense of treatment; possible personal, religious, or cultural beliefs that may contradict treatment; varying personality traits of the patient; overall denial of illness; mental disorders; or an addiction to alcohol or drugs. Also, patients may not fully understand why they need the services of the disciplines prescribed by their physician. For example, the patient may feel that they do not need the services of a SLP because they do not have any overt difficulties talking. The patients are likely unfamiliar with the full scope of the SLP's practice and may believe that they are not in need of these services. It is important, then, for the home care SLP to be aware of these possibilities for noncompliance in order to anticipate these possible issues and be prepared to address them directly when working with the patient.

Family support is critical to the success of treatment in a home care setting. However, family dynamics tend to differ across patients. Some family members may live with the patient, whereas others involved in decisions for the patient's care may live in other locations. Family members involved in the patient's care may be working during treatment visits and therefore are unavailable to participate in the rehabilitation process and post-discharge care of the patient. The family also may have unrealistic expectations for treatment or may have lower expectations for the patient's potential. These issues reinforce the need for the home care professional to communicate regularly with the patient's family regarding the patient's current abilities and potential for success in treatment. The home care professional also must communicate the importance of the family's role as the patient's main source of support.

Carryover

Because treatment duration is generally less intense than in the acute hospital or acute rehabilitation setting, implementation of carryover should be built into the home health POC as treatment is initiated. Carryover of skills learned in structured home health treatment often can be easier than in the acute setting as the patient is encouraged and challenged to use techniques, compensatory strategies, and skills in the functional home setting immediately. For optimal carryover, it is important that tasks are challenging yet that the patient feels success at the end of each session. Some techniques for carryover of skills may include:

- Have the patient keep a journal of treatment sessions and homework assignments.
- Use video recordings of sessions to document progress.
- Use charts and/or graphs to illustrate progress.
- Have family members/caregivers work with the patient outside of treatment.
- Practice skills in other environments.
- Use family members and/or friends as motivators.

Summary

- Home health care is becoming an increasingly popular setting for patients with dementia to receive services.
- Professionals working in the home health setting must be knowledgeable about the OASIS assessment, reimbursement, reassessment, and goal prioritization in order to successfully work in this environment.
- Treating a patient within their home can be very functional but also can come with a number of challenges, such as noncompliance and family considerations.
- Carryover of skills is a high priority for rehabilitation in the home setting. The treating professional must include plans for and practice of carryover of skills with both the patient and/or family/caregivers from the onset of treatment.

Authors' Note

Portions of this chapter were previously written by the authors and printed in *Perspectives on Gerontology* by the American Speech-Language-Hearing Association. Reprinted with permission from Malone, M., & Loehr, J. (2013). Home health care for adults: A tutorial for SLPs. *Perspectives on Geronology, 18*(1), 7–13. Copyright 2013 American Speech-Language-Hearing Association. All rights reserved.

References

Centers for Medicare & Medicaid Services (CMS). (2013). *Glossary*. Retrieved from http://www.medicare.gov/Homehealthcompare/Resources/Glossary.aspx

Malone, M., & Loehr, J. (2013). Home health care for adults: A tutorial for SLPs. *Perspectives on Gerontology, 18*(1), 7–13.

National Association for Home Care & Hospice. (2010). *Basic statistics about home care*. Retrieved June 30, 2013, from http://www.nahc.org/assets/1/7/10HC_Stats.pdf

Thobaben, M. (2007). Noncompliance: A challenge for home health nurses. *Home Health Care Management and Practice, 19*(5), 404–406.

Appendixes

Dementia/Aging Resource List

Alzheimer's Association
225 N. Michigan Avenue, Floor 17, Chicago, IL 60601-7633
(800) 272-3900; (866) 403-3073
http://www.alz.org

Alzheimer's Disease Education and Referral Center (ADEAR)
P.O. Box 8250, Silver Spring, MD 20907
(800) 438-4380
http://www.nia.nih.gov/alzheimers
ADEAR@alzheimers.org

Alzheimer's Foundation of America
322 Eighth Avenue, 7th Floor, New York, NY 10001
(866) AFA-8484 (866-232-8484)
http://www.alzfdn.org

AlzTalk.org
http://www.alztalk.org/

American Association of Homes and Services for the Aging (LeadingAge)
Department 5119, Washington, DC 20061
(800) 508-9442
http://www.aahsa.org

American Society on Aging
71 Stevenson Street, Suite 1450, San Francisco, CA 94105-2938
(415) 974-9600; (800) 537-9728
http://www.asaging.org

Eldercare Locator
(800) 677-1116
http://www.eldercare.gov

Family Caregiver Alliance
785 Market Street, Suite 750, San Francisco, CA 94103
(415) 434-3388; (800) 445-8106
http://www.caregiver.org
info@caregiver.org

National Academy of Elder Law Attorneys

1604 N. Country Club Road, Tucson, AZ 85716

(520) 881-4005

http://www.naela.org/

National Alliance for Caregiving

4720 Montgomery Lane, 2nd Floor, Bethesda, MD 2081

http://www.caregiving.org

NIHSeniorHealth

http://www.nihseniorhealth.gov/alzheimersdisease/toc.html

Medicare.Gov

http://www.medicare.gov

MedlinePlus

http://www.nlm.nih.gov/medlineplus/alzheimerscaregivers.html

APPENDIX B

Dementia Fact Sheet

People are living longer.

- The Centers for Disease Control (CDC) reports that the number of people aged 65 years and older is expected to increase from 35 million in 2000 to 71 million in 2030. The number of people aged 80 years and older also is expected to double, from 9.3 million in 2000 to 19.5 million in 2030 (Chapman, 2006).

The older the population gets, the more prevalent dementia becomes.

- The prevalence of dementia has been estimated to be approximately 6% to 10% of individuals aged 65 years or older; prevalence increases with age, rising from 1% to 2% among those aged 65 to 74 to 30% or more of those aged 85 or older (Chapman, 2006; Ebly, 1994; Hendrie, 1998).

Dementia affects more women than men and is more prevalent in African Americans and Hispanics.

- Of the 5.2 million people aged >65 years with AD in the United States, 3.4 million are women and 1.8 million are men.
- Older African Americans are twice as likely as older white persons to have AD and other dementias, whereas Hispanics are 1.5 times more likely than their white counterparts (Alzheimer's Association, 2012). This may be due to increased risk for high blood pressure and diabetes and reduced access to good health care.

Caregivers need care too!

- It is estimated that nearly 15 million Americans provide unpaid caregiving services to people living with dementia (Alzheimer's Association, 2012). Many of these caregivers are not well educated on dementia or how to best manage the disease and care for their loved ones.

What can we do?

- With the number of older adults growing and the possibility of the dementia population growing with it, professionals working with older adults are needed now and in the future to assist patients and caregivers in understanding dementia and how to manage it.

continues

- Ongoing education and support must be provided to these patients and caregivers, along with access to resources and referrals to services, such as speech therapy, to assist patients and families living with this disease.

Who can you contact?

- First and foremost, talk to your physician if you have concerns about dementia symptoms in yourself or a loved one.
- Agencies such as the Alzheimer's Association can help connect you to education on dementia and support services. http://www.alz.org
- Ask me!
  - Please contact me with any further questions you may have about dementia, its symptoms, or how to manage it.

    Name: _____

    Phone: _____

    Email: _____

References

Alzheimer's Association. (2012, March). Alzheimer's disease facts and figures. *Alzheimer's and Dementia: The Journal of the Alzheimer's Association, 8,* 131–168.

Chapman, D. P., Williams, S. M., Strine, T. W., Anda, R. F., & Moore, M. J. (2006, April). Dementia and its implications for public health. *Prev Chronic Dis [Serial Online].* Retrieved June 30, 2013, from http://www.cdc.gov/pcd/issues/2006/apr/05_0167.htm

Ebly, E. M., Parhad, I. M., Hogan, D. B., & Fung, T. S. Prevalence and types of dementia in the very old: Results from the Canadian Study of Health and Aging (1994). *Neurology, 44,* 1593–1600.

Hendrie, H. C. (1998). Epidemiology of dementia and Alzheimer's disease. *American Journal of Geriatric Psychiatry, 6*(2 Suppl. 1), S3–S18.

Goal Development Worksheet

Patient Name/Initials: _____

Diagnoses: _____

Payor/Insurance: _____

# of Sessions Authorized/Anticipated Length of Treatment: _____

_____

Summary of Assessment Results:

_____

_____

Patient/Caregiver Feedback:

_____

_____

_____

_____

Does Patient Agree With Need for Treatment?   Y   N

Patient Strengths/Abilities:

1.

2.

3.

Patient Personal Goals:

1.

2.

3.

Family/Caregiver Goals:

1.

2.

Is Patient Safe in Environment?   Y   N

_____

Can Patient Communicate Wants/Needs?   Y   N

_____

Is Patient Eating Safely?   Y   N

_____

Priority Areas of Treatment:

1.

2.

3.

Goals That Will Likely Lead To Early Success

1.

2.

3.

continues

Remember: Goals Should Be Measureable, Attainable, Explicit, and Functional and Include Conditions and Understandable Language.

Long-Term Goal/s:

1.

2.

3.

Short-Term Goal/s: Patient will:

1.

2.

3.

4.

5.

Caregiver Goal/s: Caregiver will:

1.

2.

3.

APPENDIX D

What Is a Swallowing Disorder?

Swallowing problems are fairly common in older adults. They can occur for many reasons, frequently it is due to a deterioration of muscle strength or coordination in the swallow mechanism. This can cause a disruption in the pathway that the food, liquid, or medication follows to get into the digestive system. At times, swallowing disorders (called dysphagia) can become serious causing a number of problems, including malnutrition, dehydration, choking, or aspiration pneumonia. The following are the most common warning signs of a swallowing problem:

1. Choking, coughing, or throat clearing while eating, drinking, or taking medications
2. Weight loss
3. Drooling
4. Food or liquid spilling from mouth during intake
5. Difficulty chewing food
6. Holding food in the cheeks
7. Avoidance of meals
8. Labored or painful swallowing
9. Runny nose during meals
10. Sensation of food or medicine 'sticking' in the throat.
11. Frequent or recurring pneumonias

People who are diagnosed with dementia are at risk to develop pneumonia as they progress into the disease process. This may be due to muscle weakness or the inability to think through the process of swallowing. The speech-language pathologist (SLP) may be able to help diagnose dysphagia and/or provide exercises and strategies to help improve swallow function and safety.

How to Talk to Someone Who Has Dementia

Dementia can affect how people form words and sentences as well as understand what is being said to them. This certainly can cause a great deal of frustration on both ends of the conversation. Here are some tips on making communication easier for the person with dementia:

1. Identify yourself. Approach the person from the front and say who you are. Keep good eye contact; if the person is sitting down, go down to that level.

2. Call the person by name. This approach helps the person get focused and pay attention.

3. Use short simple words and sentences. Too many wordy sentences can become overwhelming.

4. Speak slowly and distinctively. A slow, gentle tone in a low pitch is best.

5. Use a lot of pauses. Patiently wait for a response.

6. Repeat information or questions as needed. If the person does not respond, wait a moment then ask again.

7. Turn questions into answers. Provide the solution rather than the question. (Instead of asking, "Do you need to use the bathroom?" say, "The bathroom is right here.")

8. Turn negatives into positives. Instead of saying, "don't go here" say, "let's go here."

9. Give visual cues. To help demonstrate, point or touch the items you are referring to.

10. Avoid quizzing. One of the worst things you can ask someone with dementia is, "Do you remember when . . . ?" Try reminiscing instead.

11. Write things down. People with dementia often can read and interpret simple written words. Use this method as a supplement to conversation in order to help get your point across.

12. Treat the person with dignity and respect. Avoid talking down to the person or talking as if he or she is not in the room.

13. Watch your nonverbal language. Be aware of your feelings and attitude. A person with dementia can accurately interpret body language, facial expression, and tone of voice.

14. Avoid arguing. If the person says something you do not agree with, just move on. Arguing can create agitation.

15. Avoid criticizing or correcting. Do not tell the person that they are wrong. Instead, listen and find the meaning in what is being said. Repeat what was said if it helps to clarify the thought.

People with dementia have difficulty expressing thoughts, feelings, emotions, as well as basic wants and needs. This can create a sense of frustration and overwhelming sadness. The best approach to communication is to be patient and supportive. Offer comfort and reassurance and encourage the person to keep on communicating, whether it is verbal or nonverbal communication.

Creating a Safe Environment

As the dementia progresses, it is common for the person with dementia to lose the ability to make good decisions, plan ahead, and sometimes even understand consequences. There are many safety hazards that can be found in the home. These hazards do not actually exist until someone develops dementia and is unable to demonstrate sound judgment. The following are tips for creating a safe living environment for someone who suffers from dementia:

1. Remove throw rugs, bath mats, and door mats. These are one of the most common causes of falls in the home.

2. Move furniture so that there is a clear path throughout the home.

3. Put all household poisons in a locked cabinet.

4. Arrange locks to exterior doors (that may open to hazardous areas like busy streets) on the inside and out of reach.

5. Put alarms on exterior doors to prevent wandering.

6. Remove knobs on stoves/oven when not in use.

7. Put hazardous household appliances and power tools out of sight.

8. Keep all medicine in a locked cabinet. Keep an updated list of medicines available and easy to access should an emergency arise.

9. Keep clutter to a minimum.

10. Change light bulbs to higher wattage to accommodate vision deficits.

11. Keep candy and sweets out of reach and out of sight.

12. Avoid excess noise and stimulation (especially if you want to have a conversation!).

13. Keep the car keys hidden and the car doors locked.

14. Pets can be a tripping hazard. Determine if pets need to be closely monitored and tethered while in the home.

15. Mop up spills immediately. This includes excess water in the bathroom after a shower or bath. Visual deficits make it hard to avoid slips on wet surfaces.

16. Install hand rails in the bathroom. Many falls happen when people try to use the towel rack to get up from the toilet.

17. Consider using an emergency call system installed in your home and teach your loved one to use this early on.

What Activities Are Best for a Person With Dementia?

Quality time spent with your loved one or friend may seem uncomfortable as conversation is difficult and often times getting out to do activities is difficult, if not exhausting. There are a number of activities that you and the person with dementia can engage in together to make your time together meaningful. Here are a few tips to follow to ensure success:

1. Keep the person's skill level and interest in mind. (Did they play the piano? Were they a painter?)

2. Pay attention to what this person enjoys. (If they do not like cooking, stay away from the kitchen.)

3. Provide activities that do not require instruction. (Put a rolling pin and cookie dough in front of someone, generally they know what to do.)

4. Be aware of physical limitations. (If they have a tremor or weakness, avoid tasks that require fine motor skills. For example, writing, drawing, and painting.)

5. Make sure the outcome is enjoyment not achievement. (Was it fun? Who cares what it looks like in the end!)

6. Make the activity meaningful and functional to daily living activities. (Household chores are relatively easy to understand and execute. They provide a great sense of satisfaction in the end.)

7. Relate the activity to past work or hobby. (i.e., A secretary may enjoy filing. A fisherman may enjoy tying flies.)

8. Find a time of day that is optimal for the activity. (Do not initiate an activity right before bedtime.)

9. Be flexible. (Let them do it "their way.")

10. Offer support and supervision. Assist with difficult parts of the task. (i.e., In building a birdhouse, perhaps you help with using tools or applying glue.)

11. Let the individual know that he/she is needed in the task. Stress a sense of purpose. (Let the person know what they are doing is important and meaningful. Let them know how important it is to spend time with you.)

12. Do not criticize or correct. (It does not matter if it is wrong.)

13. Encourage self-expression (Remember that speech/language may be impaired; music or art can take the place of expressing emotion verbally.)

14. Involve conversation. (Sometimes focusing on an activity makes it easier for speech/language.)

continues

15. Substitute an activity for a behavior. (Painting, listening to music, or clipping coupons can be relaxing.)

16. Try again later. (If the task becomes frustrating, overwhelming, or causes negative emotions, it is time to stop and walk away from the task.)

Tips for Preventing Weight Loss

It is common for the person with dementia to lose weight as the disease progresses. The reasons for weight loss are numerous. Your loved one may be suffering from a loss of appetite due to depression, medication interaction, or a change in taste/smell sensations. They also may begin to lose the cognitive ability to feed themselves or suffer from some changes in the oral cavity making chewing or swallowing uncomfortable. Here are some tips for improving appetite and keeping your loved one well hydrated:

1. Make sure that the food is easily seen on the plate. Use plates that are brightly colored and make sure that the food is contrasted. Ensure that there is adequate lighting at the dinner table.

2. Do not overload the plate with food. It is easy for your loved one to get overwhelmed by too much food creating a loss of appetite. If possible, offer one portion at a time in separate bowls or plates.

3. Create a soothing and pleasant eating environment. Eliminate excess noise that is distracting. Turn off the television and turn on some soothing music instead. Keep the conversation to a minimum, especially if there is a risk for choking.

4. Spice it up! Taste and smell sensations tend to get dull as we age. Adding extra sugar to some foods can help. Try using agave nectar, chocolate sauce, or maple syrup on top of the entrees (yes, on top of the steak, pasta, chicken, etc.). You may be surprised that this tastes really good to your loved one!

5. Make it easy to chew. Sometimes when chewing or swallowing gets difficult, mealtime can become a negative experience creating an avoidance behavior. Make sure the food is prepared so that it is easy to chew and swallow. Observe your loved one while he/she is eating. Does it look like they are struggling? They may not be able to verbally tell you that they are having trouble.

6. Offer a lot of liquids during the meal. This will help keep your loved one hydrated and also help get the foods down as well. Losing the sensation of thirst (or being able to identify thirst) is common as we age. Consequently, dehydration is common.

7. Stimulate appetite with fragrances. The scent of geranium will stimulate appetite. If you are able to find geranium scented oil or lotion, use it on a hot moist towel as a face and hand wash prior to meals. Try baking cookies, cakes, or pastries right before a meal. The scent of fresh-baked cookies stimulates the appetite.

8. Do not make mealtime a struggle. Arguing or force-feeding your loved one will not help to improve appetite or increase intake.

continues

9. Offer six small meals a day instead of three large meals.

10. Stick to the favorites! Your loved one may enjoy the same food every day for months. Even though it might seem horrible to us to have limited variety, to your loved one that familiar homemade dish may be very comforting.

11. Try finger foods. It may be easier for your loved one to eat with his/her hands as utensils have become confusing. At the same time, some finger foods may be confusing such as breakfast tacos or burritos (especially if the contents fall onto the plate).

12. Do not rush! Sometimes mealtime can take a lot longer for the person who has dementia.

13. Offer small snacks during the day.

14. Provide choices. It can be very satisfying for your loved one to be given a choice (when they have very little opportunity for choice in their lives). Just by offering a choice between water or milk, salt or pepper, mustard or ketchup can be very pleasing. If your loved one cannot verbally state what they want, perhaps they can point or look in the direction of their choice.

Index

Note: Page numbers in **bold** reference non-text material.